Atlas of Clinical Imaging and Anatomy of the Equine Head

To my wonderful wife and family – who make everything I do possible, fun and worthwhile – Jan, Buddy, Katie, Jana, Eli.

Larry Kimberlin

To my amazing, strong, and beautiful wife, Emily. A lover of all creatures great and small.

Alex zur Linden

To my late husband, Dub, and my children Brett and Cathy – your support has been instrumental in anything I have accomplished.

Lynn Ruoff

Atlas of Clinical Imaging and Anatomy of the Equine Head

Larry Kimberlin, DVM, FAVD, CVPP

Alex zur Linden, DVM, DACVR

Lynn Ruoff, DVM

WILEY Blackwell

This edition first published 2017 © 2017 by John Wiley & Sons, Inc.

Editorial Offices
1606 Golden Aspen Drive, Suites 103 and 104, Ames, Iowa 50010, USA
The Atrium, Southern Gate, Chichester, West Sussex, PO19 8SQ, UK
9600 Garsington Road, Oxford, OX4 2DQ, UK

For details of our global editorial offices, for customer services and for information about how to apply for permission to reuse the copyright material in this book please see our website at www.wiley.com/wiley-blackwell.

Library of Congress Cataloging-in-Publication Data

Names: Kimberlin, Larry, 1956– author. | Zur Linden, Alex, 1979– author. | Ruoff, Lynn, 1951– author.
Title: Atlas of clinical imaging and anatomy of the equine head / Larry Kimberlin, Alex zur Linden, Lynn Ruoff.
Description: Ames, Iowa : John Wiley & Sons, Inc., 2017. | Includes bibliographical references and index.
Identifiers: LCCN 2016023788 (print) | LCCN 2016030763 (ebook) | ISBN 9781118988978 (cloth) |
    ISBN 9781118988985 (pdf) | ISBN 9781118988992 (epub)
Subjects: LCSH: Horses–Anatomy–Atlases. | Head–Anatomy–Atlases. | Head–Imaging–Atlases. |
    MESH: Horses–anatomy & histology | Head–anatomy & histology | Diagnostic Imaging–veterinary |
    Anatomy, Veterinary | Atlases
Classification: LCC SF765 .K56 2017 (print) | LCC SF765 (ebook) | NLM SF 765 | DDC 636.1/0891–dc23
LC record available at https://lccn.loc.gov/2016023788

A catalogue record for this book is available from the British Library.

Wiley also publishes its books in a variety of electronic formats. Some content that appears in print may not be available in electronic books.

Set in 9.5/12 pt MinionPro by SPi Global, Pondicherry, India
Printed and bound in Singapore by Markono Print Media Pte Ltd

1 2017

Contents

Introduction: General Presentation of Atlas

The equine head is a clinically important part of the equine patient. It provides residence to the most important structure of any patient – the brain. The brain is the control center for all activities of its host. The head also contains the primary structural components of four of the five senses (*sight, hearing, taste, smell,* and *touch*).

Major components of all the major body systems are present here as well:

- the brain and cranial nerves
- the entry point of food for the digestive system
- the entry point of air for the respiratory system
- the activating and stimulating precursors of the endocrine system
- the vascular system is well represented, as well as the integumentary system.

As such, the head has long been clinically and surgically important for the equine practitioner. Radiography has been the gold standard for diagnosing and treating pathologic conditions related to the head. Two-dimensional plain film radiographs have been instrumental in the clinician's armamentarium, but technologic advances in cross-sectional imaging have now become the gold standard for diagnosis and treatment planning of trauma, neurologic, dental, and sinus/airway disease. Improvements in technology and decreased costs have made cross-sectional imaging more accessible to the practitioner. It is the authors' opinion that in the near future, cross-sectional imaging will become standard of care for diagnosis of many equine diseases.

It was with this thought in mind that the idea for this atlas was born. Until now, there has been no comprehensive comparative atlas for structures of the head. The three-plane cross-sectional composition of the cadaver pictures allows the student and clinician to view structures of the head that may not be readily visible by dissection alone. The multiplanar preparation allows direct comparison of the structures with the corresponding imaging modalities of CT and MRI scanning.

The authors have attempted to identify the clinically important structures of the head to use as a reference for understanding anatomy and pathology, and as a surgical reference. The anatomy has been labeled with the help of anatomical atlases and peer-reviewed scientific journals. Each structure is identified in the cadaver and each imaging modality (if visible) for comparison. A legend is included for each image that identifies the location and direction of the slice. An index key for each structure is present on each image with further designation of the body system.

1. Bones of the head
2. Oral and dental structures
3. Nasal and sinus structures
4. Larynx, pharynx, and guttural pouches
5. Ophthalmic structures
6. Auricular structures
7. Brain and nervous system
8. Vascular anatomy
9. Muscles
10. Glandular structures – lymph and salivary

It is the authors' sincere hope that this atlas will aid students and clinicians as a study and clinical guide to better understand the anatomy of the equine head, as part of our mission to help our patients and their owners by treatment of pathologic processes encountered in daily practice.

Larry Kimberlin DVM, FAVD, CVPP
Alex zur Linden DVM, DACVR
Lynn Ruoff DVM

CHAPTER 1
Overview of CT and MRI of the Equine Head

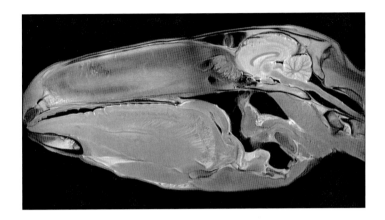

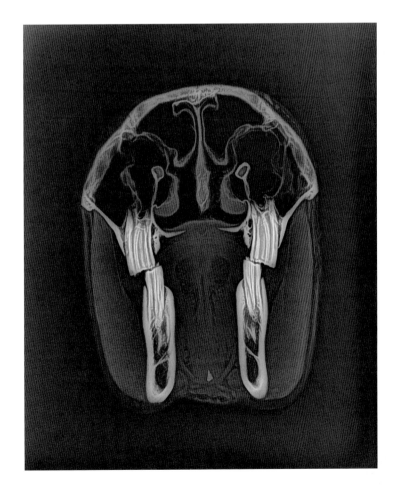

Atlas of Clinical Imaging and Anatomy of the Equine Head, First Edition. Larry Kimberlin, Alex zur Linden and Lynn Ruoff.

The diagnosis of conditions affecting the equine head is challenging for the veterinary practitioner due to its large size, complex anatomy, and the multitude of different tissues present and thus the large number of potential disease processes. Disease processes of the teeth include caries, periodontal disease, tooth root abscess, tooth fracture, dentigerous cysts, and malocclusion to name a few [1]. The tongue can be affected by trauma, infection, or neoplasia. The nasal passages and paranasal sinuses are important parts of the equine head that can be the site of sinusitis, ethmoid hematomas, cysts, or neoplasia. The diverticulum of the auditory tube (guttural pouch) can develop fungal granulomas, empyema, blood clots, or tympany. Laryngeal hemiplegia, dorsal displacement of the soft palate, epiglottic entrapment, rostral displacement of the palatopharyngeal arches, arytenoid chondritis, and pharyngeal narrowing can affect the pharyngeal region [2]. Other tissues in the head such as the lymph nodes and salivary glands can be affected by infectious or non-infectious inflammation, or neoplasia. The brain can be affected by trauma, bleeding, infarction, neoplasms, cholesterinic granulomas, ventriculomegaly (hydrocephalus), and infection (meningitis or meningoencephalitis). Trauma to the head can result in fractures of the calvarium, mandible, temporomandibular joint, basisphenoid bone, and nuchal crest of the occipital bone. Although uncommon in horses, neoplasia that can be found in the head includes melanoma, adenocarcinoma or rhabdomyosarcoma of the tongue, lacrimal gland adenocarcinoma and ophthalmic tumors associated with the eye, and multicentric lymphoma affecting the lymph nodes in the head [2]. The hyoid bones can be affected by fractures or temporohyoid osteoarthropathy. The eyes and ears are also prone to a variety of pathological conditions. Many of these conditions can be diagnosed on physical examination; however, many require further diagnostics.

Diagnostic imaging of the equine head is most commonly done via radiography (Figure 1) or endoscopy. Routine radiographic examination can include orthogonal projections of the area of interest, oblique projections of the dental arcades or temporomandibular joints and intraoral projections for the rostral mandible/maxilla. Due to the size of the adult head and the limited size of the X-ray cassette or imaging plate, multiple radiographs are needed to image the entire head, although this is not routinely performed in clinical practice. Radiographs offer superior spatial resolution compared to more advanced imaging options; however, due to the superimposition of anatomy, lesion localization can be quite challenging using radiography. The anatomy of the head is complex and radiographs

(b)

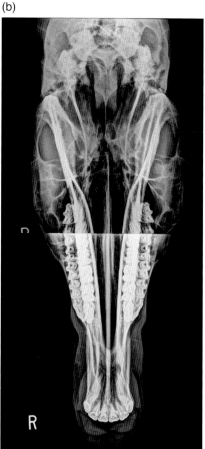

(a)

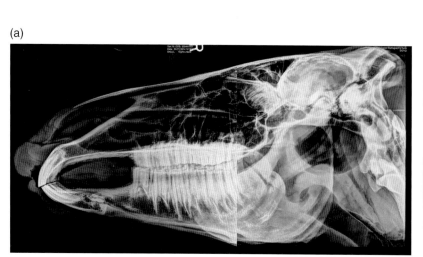

Figure 1 A lateral (a) and dorsoventral radiograph (b) of the head from an older adult equine cadaver that was used in the making of this book. Two radiographs are spliced together to create each image of the whole head. These radiographs demonstrate the excellent contrast between the air-filled nasal passages, paranasal sinuses and guttural pouches, and the mineral opaque bones and teeth. The soft tissues are difficult to differentiate unless they are surrounded by gas or bone.

do not provide adequate contrast of the soft tissues of the head. Radiographic anatomy has been thoroughly described elsewhere and is outside the scope of this book.

A computed tomography (CT) unit consists of a high-powered X-ray tube mounted in a circular gantry across from a detector array. The gantry is able to rotate around the patient using slip-ring technology so it is not tethered electronically to the rest of the unit. As the gantry rotates, the patient moves either into or out of the gantry as the X-rays are absorbed, scattered, or pass through the patient. The X-rays that reach the detector array are used to construct an image.

For digital radiographs, the attenuation of the X-rays results in a two-dimensional image involving multiple pixels. CT uses a similar method to display an image by converting a volume of tissue to a three-dimensional pixel called a voxel. CT will determine the average linear attenuation coefficient of X-rays for each voxel in a patient at a particular location [3]. Each voxel can be given a quantifiable number in terms of its gray scale, termed a Hounsfield unit (HU). As a reference, pure water has a HU of 0 and air is −1000 HU. Adipose tissue can vary from −30 to −80 HU, soft tissues +30 to +220, while bone and iodinated contrast media can be close to +2000 to +3000. Each voxel is then interpreted as a pixel when displayed as a two-dimensional CT image.

Most CT images are reconstructed in an axial plane. If the depth of the slice thickness (z-direction of the voxel) is the same as the size of the pixel (x and y directions), then the voxel is considered isotropic, or near isotropic if it is similar in size. Isotropic voxels allow for high-resolution reconstructions of the CT dataset into multiple different planes. These reconstructions allow one to view the anatomy in different planes to identify the extent of a disease process or to better visualize the "three-dimensional" (3D) anatomy using a two-dimensional interface. Isotropic voxels can also be used to produce high-resolution reconstructions that appear three-dimensional, even though they are still a two-dimensional image. This is demonstrated in Figure 2c and d, where a 3D reconstruction can be useful to get an overall look at the scanned anatomical structures.

Computed tomography images are reconstructed from a very large collection of voxels (raw image data), each with its own Hounsfield unit and location in space. The computer uses an algorithm or filter to adjust how each pixel looks on a two-dimensional image and this algorithm can be modified to alter the spatial resolution and contrast differences of different tissues. The primary two algorithms used in this book are referred to generically as a bone filter or algorithm and a soft tissue filter or algorithm. The bone algorithm has a higher spatial resolution and the bone and teeth are seen in gray with well-defined edges, whereas all the soft tissues are homogenously gray. The soft tissue algorithm has a reduced spatial resolution but the contrast of the soft tissues is more noticeable, and the bone and teeth are completely white.

The appearance of the CT images can be adjusted by the viewer for either algorithm using the window width/window level adjustment function found on all image viewing systems. The window width (WW) is the range of displayed Hounsfield units. The window level (WL) is the Hounsfield unit in the center of the window width. In this book, the bone algorithm is shown in a bone window, with a WW of ~3500 and a WL of ~650. The soft tissue algorithm is shown in a soft tissue window, with a WW of ~500 and a WL of ~70. So, for the bone setting a wide window of 3500 densities allows for a lot of different densities to be displayed, centered on 650 HU (+4150 to −2850 HU). For the soft tissue setting, a short window width of 500 is used, centered at 70 HU, near the density of the soft tissues of the head (+570 HU to −430 HU). Anything with a higher density than these ranges will be white, and anything with a lower density will be black. Everything in between will be a shade of gray. For viewing the brain, an even smaller window is needed to assess the difference between gray and white matter. These images were not used to depict the brain anatomy in this book due to space requirements. Figure 3 demonstrates the brain WW/WL in a horse with cholesterinic granulomas and ventriculomegaly.

Magnetic resonance imaging (MRI) is another cross-sectional imaging modality, but unlike CT, it does not involve ionizing radiation Instead, MRI uses nuclear magnetic resonance, the absorption and release of energy from the nucleus of an atom when placed in a strong magnetic field. Although different atoms can be used for imaging, in living tissue primarily hydrogen is used as it has the largest magnetic moment and is in greatest abundance in water and fat [3]. The nucleus of the hydrogen atom, which consists of a proton, is the focus for generating the MR signal. The patient is placed on the MRI table with the body part of interest to be imaged within a coil. This coil allows radiofrequency signals to be emitted, received, or both. This radiofrequency energy is absorbed by the protons in the body and emitted at certain rates (T2 and T1 relaxation). There are multiple different types of MR sequences that can be performed, and for the most part they are related to timing differences of the emitted energy from the protons, or relaxation times. These sequences include T2 weighted, T1 weighted, T2* weighted, proton density (PD), and inversion recovery (fat or fluid suppression).

T2-weighted sequences are primarily used to identify pathology such as inflammation or edema. The T2 relaxation between different tissues allows for the excellent contrast seen between cerebrospinal fluid (CSF), gray and white matter of the brain, and fat (Figure 4a,d). With T1-weighted sequences, the contrast between the CSF, gray and white matter, and the fat is reduced, but the resolution and anatomic detail are improved. Also, contrast media (gadolinium based) can be administered intravenously and assessed with T1-weighted imaging (Figure 4c) to increase lesion conspicuousness. This contrast medium reduces the T1 relaxation time, resulting in increased signal intensity on T1-weighted sequences [4]. This increased signal is present within blood vessels and in tissues that have an increased blood flow. In brain tissue, this would result from a break down of the blood–brain barrier.

Proton density contrast weighting depends on the difference in magnetized protons within different tissues [3]. This sequence results in proton-dense tissues such as CSF having a high (bright) signal intensity. This leads to the highest overall

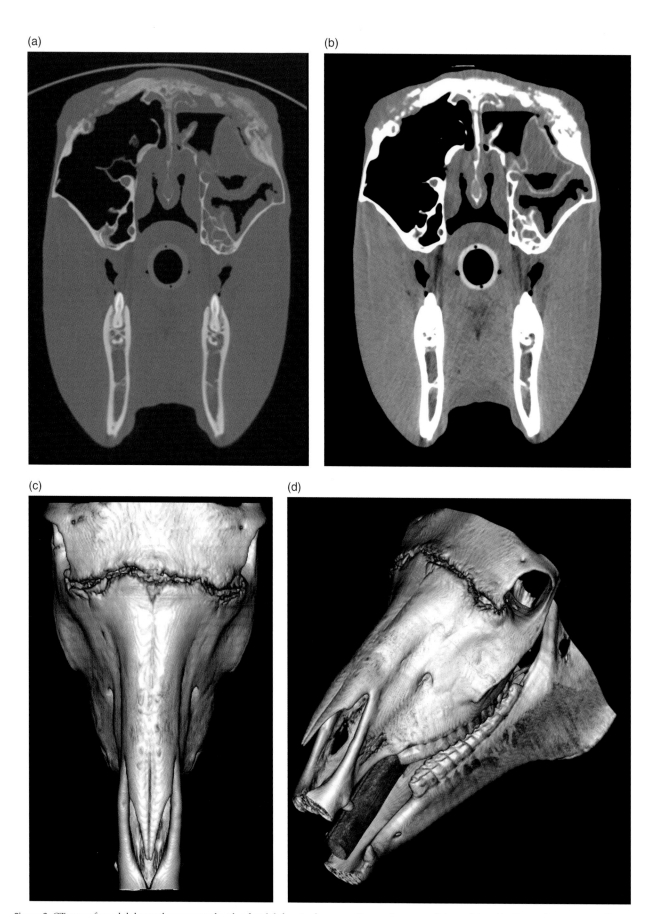

Figure 2 CT scan of an adult horse that presented with a facial deformity from an unknown trauma and signs of sinusitis. The patient was imaged in dorsal recumbency for the CT scan. (a,b) Transverse images at the level of the fracture in a bone filter and window (a) and a soft tissue filter and window (b), demonstrating thickened and irregular margins of the frontal, nasal, and lacrimal bones. Fluid is also noted in the conchofrontal sinus and caudally displaced ventral conchal sinus. The lining of the sinuses is thickened, consistent with sinusitis. (c,d) "Three-dimensional" reconstructions of the CT dataset with a dorsal view (c) and left dorsolateral view (d) of the skull. These images help to get an overall look at the bones of the skull and to determine that this deformity was likely caused by a concussive trauma to a sharp linear object, such as the corner of a beam or post. The displacement of the ventral conchal sinus and concha caused by the trauma caused narrowing of the conchomaxillary opening that impeded drainage, resulting in the sinusitis.

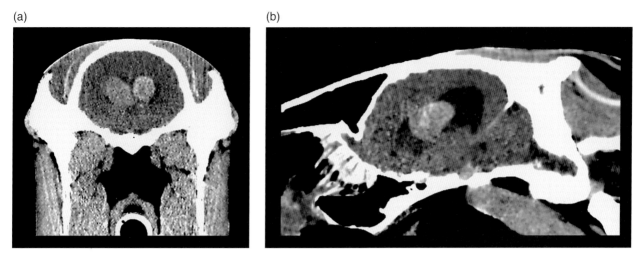

Figure 3 Transverse (a) and sagittal (b) reconstructions of a CT scan of an adult horse that presented with a history of seizures. The WW is 83 and WL is 27. Within each lateral ventricle is an ovoid, faintly mineral-dense structure arising from the choroid plexus. There is also fluid distension of the lateral ventricles, consistent with an obstruction to CSF outflow. These mineralized structures are consistent with cholesterinic granulomas causing an obstructive hydrocephalus.

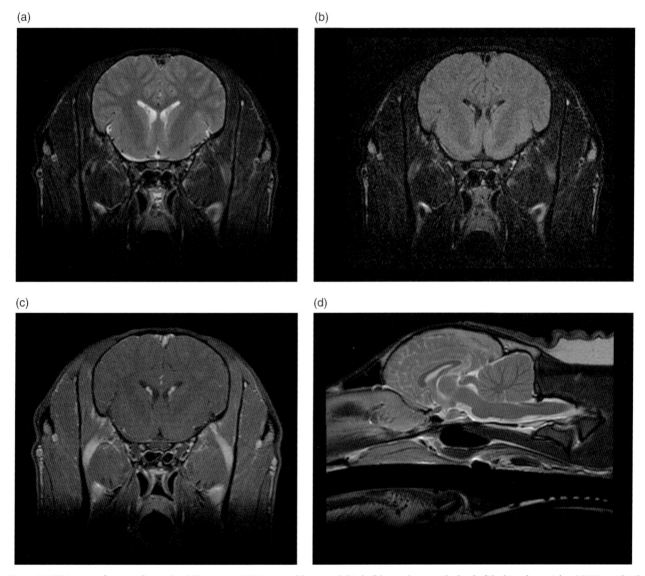

Figure 4 MRI images of a young horse. (a–c) Transverse MR images of the rostral third of the cerebrum at the level of the lateral ventricles. (a) T2-weighted sequence. (b) FLAIR sequence. (c) T1-weighted sequence plus contrast administration (gadolinium) and fat saturation. Note the fluid suppression of the CSF on the FLAIR sequence (b) in the lateral ventricles when compared to (a). (d) Sagittal plane, T2-weighted sequence of the brain on midline. In (c), there is contrast enhancement of the choroid plexus in the lateral ventricles, and the blood vessels ventral to the brain.

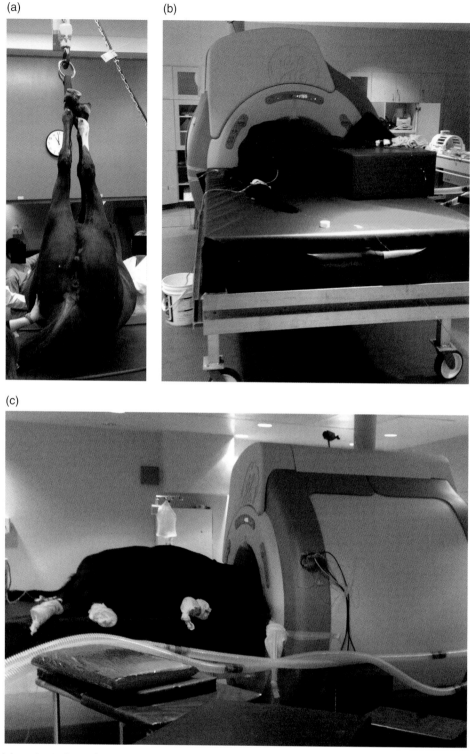

Figure 5 (a) An adult horse is raised onto the MRI table with hobbles placed around the feet and a ceiling hoist. The table is then rolled into the MRI suite, the wheels locked, and the patient moved forward into the magnet by sliding it across the padded table (b,c). (b) View from the MRI control room of the horse in the magnet. (c) Side view from the entry door of the horse in the magnet.

signal intensity and signal-to-noise ratio, while the image contrast is slightly reduced [3]. Inversion recovery is another type of MR sequence, and can null the signal from either fluid (fluid attenuation inversion recovery or FLAIR) or fat (short-tau inversion recovery or STIR). The FLAIR sequence is useful to differentiate pure fluid from proteinaceous fluid, and to better define the margins of a fluid-filled space or pocket. The STIR sequence is useful to identify pathology (inflammation, edema) without mistaking it for hyperintense fat. The last common type of sequence is a T2*-weighted sequence. This is susceptible to magnetic field inhomogeneities, and is particularly useful to identify hemoglobin breakdown products. A

(a)

(b)

(c)

(d)

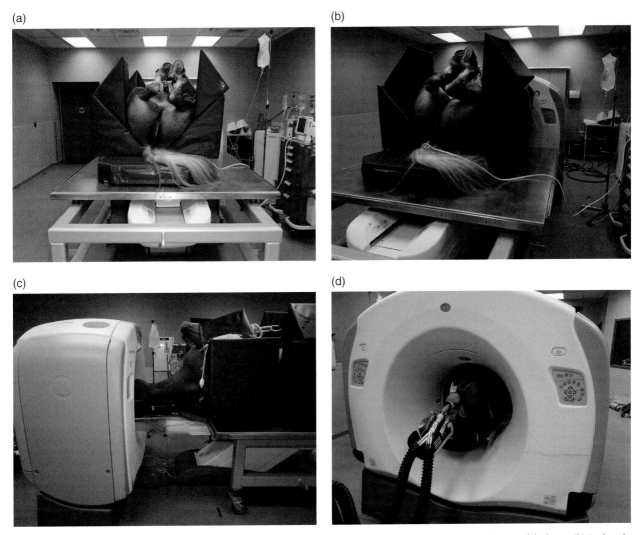

Figure 6 An adult horse has been hoisted onto the large animal CT table and positioned in dorsal recumbency. (a) Back view of the horse. (b) Back and side view of the horse. (c) Side view of the horse. (d) Front view of the scanner with the horse intubated and connected to the anesthetic equipment.

more in-depth discussion of the physics of MRI and these sequences is beyond the scope of this book and can be learned elsewhere [3].

The proton density sequence images were chosen for this book based on the esthetics of the images when compared to T1- and T2-weighted images, the image contrast of the brain, and the adequate depiction of all the different anatomical structures in the head.

Equine CT and MRI scans require proper facilities and equipment for holding and moving the animals. At our facility, we have two different large animal tables. The table for MRI is non-ferromagnetic so it can be used in the MRI suite (Figure 5). A ceiling hoist is needed to move the patient from the induction stall to the table with the use of hobbles (Figure 5a). Large soft pads are needed under the patient to prevent muscle damage. The patient is moved so the area of interest (rostral or caudal portion of the head) is placed in the middle of the magnet (iso-center) (Figure 5b,c). The MRI large animal table does not move during scanning.

The large animal CT table is different from the MRI table as it connects directly to the smaller CT bed underneath, allowing the table to move during scanning. Patients are often imaged in dorsal recumbency, with the area of interest (rostral or caudal head) in the CT gantry (Figure 6). As the scan starts, the patient is moved out of the scanner until the region of interest is scanned. Intravenous iodinated contrast medium can be administered and the scan repeated.

Indications for performing CT versus MRI

At our institution, equine head CT scans are more frequently performed than MRI scans. These are typically used to evaluate the teeth and sinuses, and for fractures following trauma. CT allows for excellent visualization of the tooth roots, clear delineation of the nasal passages and paranasal sinuses, and partial visualization of the brain and soft tissues. MRI provides much better contrast of the brain and soft tissues of the head. A major limitation to doing an MRI of the brain of a horse is that the patient likely has neurological signs. This would also apply to neurological patients presenting for a CT scan of the head. Recovery of a neurological horse can be problematic and result in head trauma or fractured limbs. MRI has been reported to be more sensitive to physiological processes of the head and central nervous system than CT, and has been successfully used as a neurodiagnostic modality in horses [5].

Both CT and MRI require general anesthesia and are expensive, with a limited number of institutions having the ability to image large animals with CT and/or MRI. The risk of the patient undergoing general anesthesia for a CT or MRI needs to be less than the potential benefit of the information gained from such a scan. For those patients that do undergo a cross-sectional imaging scan at your facility, this book should serve as a quick and useful reference to help you better understand the complex anatomy of the equine head.

Notes

The dorsal and sagittal MRI images have been stitched together using Siemens Composer software. This is not used for diagnostic purposes, but does give a better perspective of the anatomy in relation to the whole head and is very useful for the purposes of this book.

The sequence parameters for the PD MRI sequences were: TE 28, TR 6174.8, FS 3, 4.4 mm slice thickness. CT and MRI scans of the equine cadaver heads were performed by Animal Imaging, Irving, Texas.

References

1 O'Brien RT, Biller DS (1998) Dental imaging. *Veterinary Clinics of North America Equine Practitioner*, **14**, 259.
2 Reed SM, Bayly WM, Sellon DC (2010) *Equine Internal Medicine*, 3rd edn. Saunders Elsevier, St Louis.
3 Bushberg JT, Seibert JA, Leidholdt EM, Boone JM (2012) *The Essential Physics of Medical Imaging*, 3rd edn. Lippincott Williams and Wilkins, Philadelphia.
4 Saveraid TC, Judy CE (2012) Use of intravenous gadolinium contrast in equine magnetic resonance imaging. *Veterinary Clinics of North America, Equine Practitioner*, **28**, 617–636.
5 Ferrell EA, Gavin PR, Tucker RL, Sellon DC, Hines MT (2002) Magnetic resonance for evaluation of neurologic disease in 12 horses. *Veterinary Radiology and Ultrasound*, **43** (6), 510–516.

CHAPTER 2
Clinical and Surgical Anatomy of the Equine Head: Transverse Sections

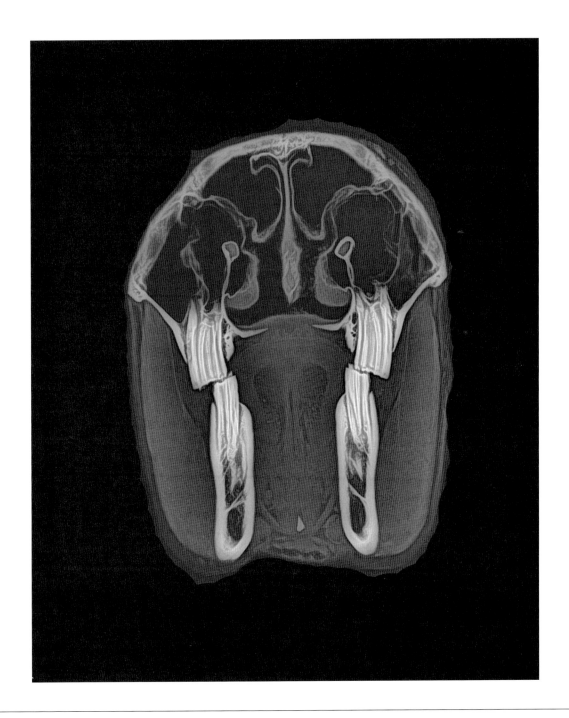

Atlas of Clinical Imaging and Anatomy of the Equine Head, First Edition. Larry Kimberlin, Alex zur Linden and Lynn Ruoff.
© 2017 John Wiley & Sons, Inc. Published 2017 by John Wiley & Sons, Inc.

T1

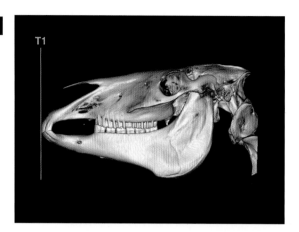

1. **Bones of the head**
2. Oral and dental structures
3. **Nasal and sinus structures**
4. Larynx, pharynx, and guttural pouches
5. **Ophthalmic structures**
6. **Auricular structures**
7. Brain and nervous system
8. **Vascular anatomy**
9. Muscles
10. **Glandular structures – lymph and salivary**

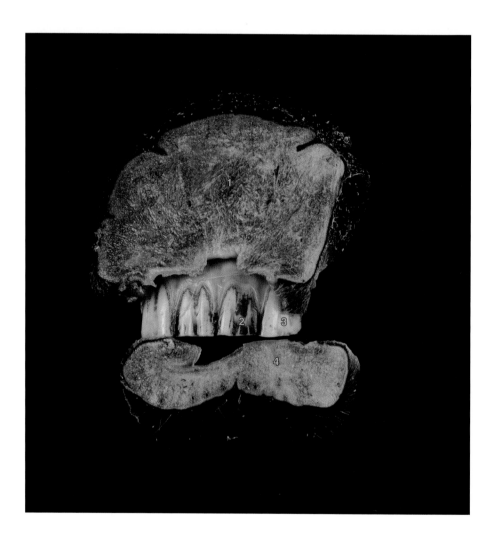

1 Labium superioris (upper lip)
2 Tooth number 201 (left upper central incisor)
3 Tooth number 202 (left upper intermediate incisor)
4 Labium inferioris (lower lip)

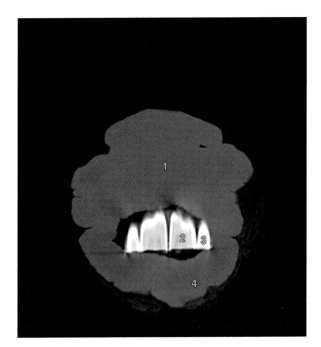

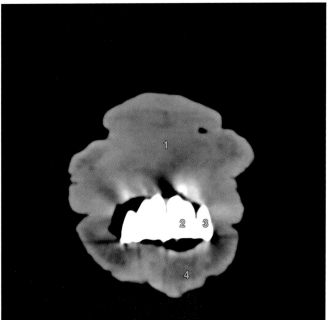

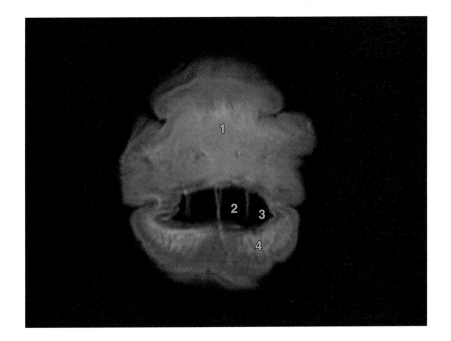

T2

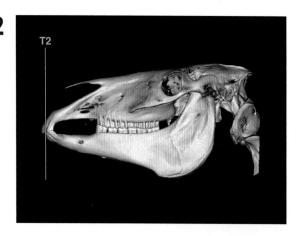

1. **Bones of the head**
2. Oral and dental structures
3. **Nasal and sinus structures**
4. Larynx, pharynx, and guttural pouches
5. Ophthalmic structures
6. Auricular structures
7. Brain and nervous system
8. **Vascular anatomy**
9. Muscles
10. **Glandular structures – lymph and salivary**

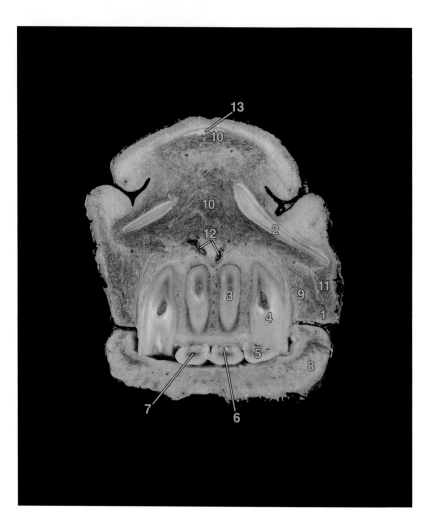

1 Labium superioris (superior lip)
2 Cornu (horn) of the alar cartilage (left)
3 Tooth 201 (left superior central incisor)
4 Tooth 202 (left superior intermediate incisor)
5 Tooth 302 (left inferior central incisor)

6 "Enamel spot" of tooth 301 (left inferior central incisor)
7 Pulp of tooth 401 (right inferior central incisor)
8 Labium inferioris (inferior lip)
9 Minor labial salivary glands

10 Apical naris dilatator m.
11 Orbicularis oris m.
12 Terminal branch of the major palatine a.
13 Levator labii superior tendon

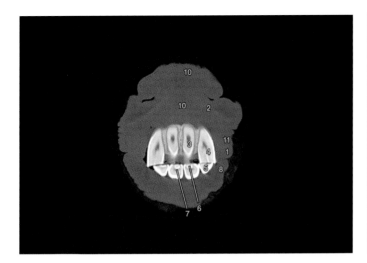

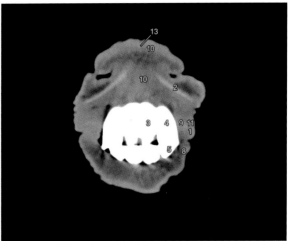

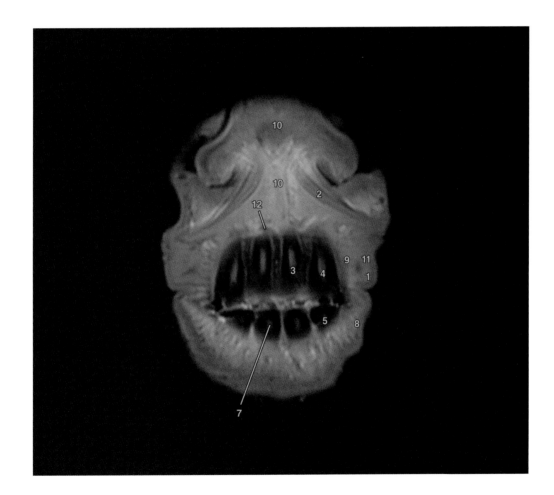

T3

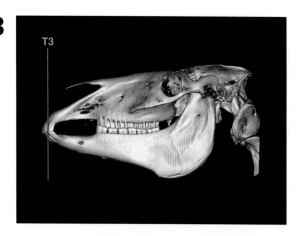

1. **Bones of the head**
2. Oral and dental structures
3. **Nasal and sinus structures**
4. Larynx, pharynx, and guttural pouches
5. **Ophthalmic structures**
6. **Auricular structures**
7. Brain and nervous system
8. **Vascular anatomy**
9. Muscles
10. **Glandular structures – lymph and salivary**

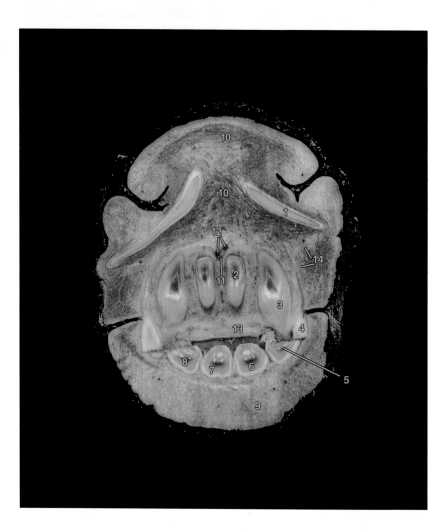

1 Cornu (horn) of the alar cartilage	5 Tooth 302 (left inferior intermediate incisor)	10 Apical naris dilatator m.
2 Pulp cavity of tooth 201 (left superior central incisor)	6 Tooth 301 (left inferior central incisor)	**11 Interincisive canal**
3 Tooth 202 (left superior intermediate incisor)	7 Tooth 401 (right inferior central incisor)	**12 Terminal branch of the major palatine a.**
4 Tooth 203 (left superior corner incisor)	8 Tooth 402 (right inferior intermediate incisor)	13 Body of the incisive bone (rostral hard palate)
	9 Labia inferioris (inferior lip)	**14 Minor labial salivary glands**

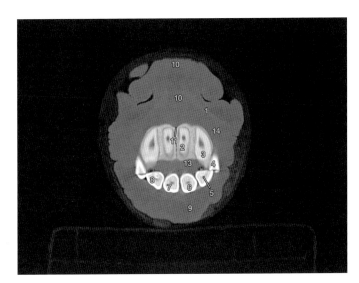

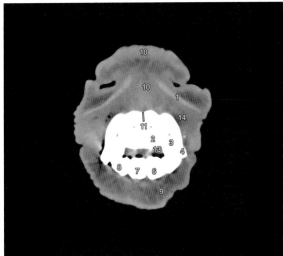

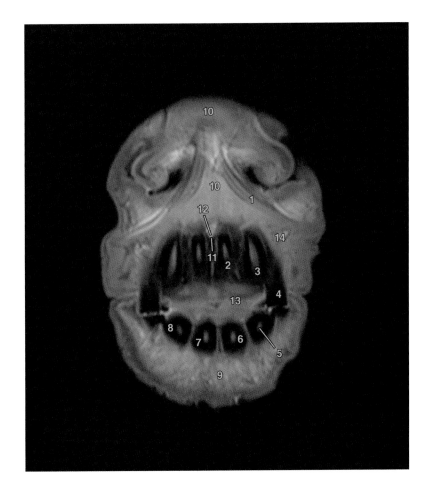

T4

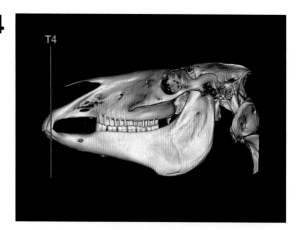

1. **Bones of the head**
2. Oral and dental structures
3. **Nasal and sinus structures**
4. Larynx, pharynx, and guttural pouches
5. Ophthalmic structures
6. **Auricular structures**
7. Brain and nervous system
8. **Vascular anatomy**
9. Muscles
10. **Glandular structures – lymph and salivary**

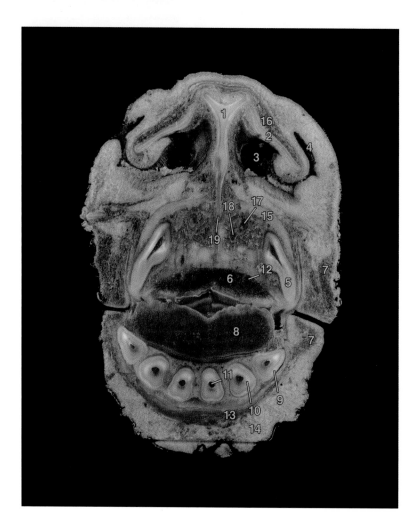

1 Nasal septum	**6 Stratum cavernosum of the hard palate**	**11 Tooth 301 (left inferior central incisor)**
2 Alar cartilage	7 Orbicularis oris m.	**12 Buccal salivary gland**
3 Vestibule of the nasal cavity	8 Intrinsic muscles of the tongue	**13 Major palatine a.**
4 Nasal diverticulum ("false nostril")	9 Tooth 303 (left inferior corner incisor)	14 Rugae of hard palate
5 Tooth 203 (left superior corner incisor)	10 Tooth 302 (left inferior intermediate incisor)	

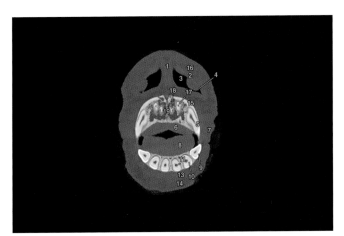

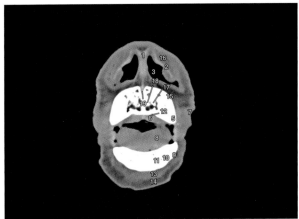

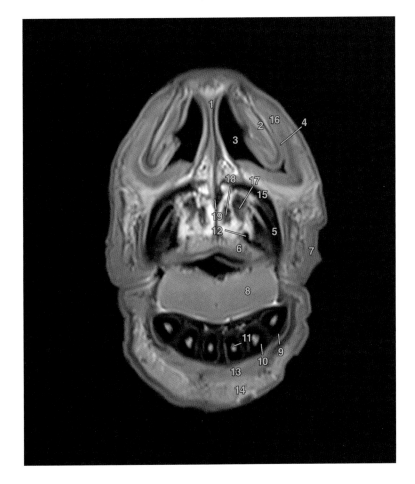

T5

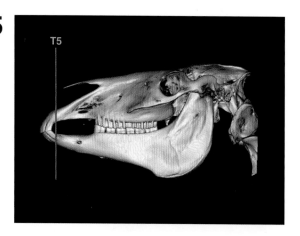

1. **Bones of the head**
2. **Oral and dental structures**
3. **Nasal and sinus structures**
4. Larynx, pharynx, and guttural pouches
5. **Ophthalmic structures**
6. **Auricular structures**
7. Brain and nervous system
8. **Vascular anatomy**
9. Muscles
10. **Glandular structures – lymph and salivary**

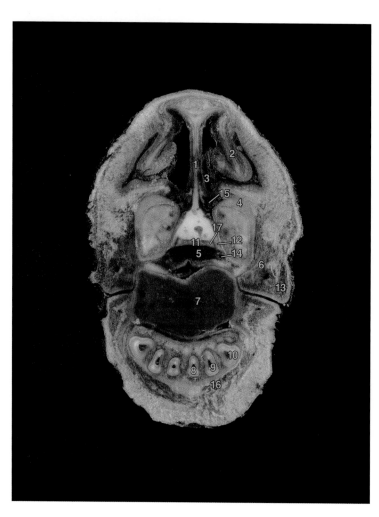

1 Nasal septum
2 Lamina (plate) of the alar cartilage
3 Vestibule of the nasal cavity
4 Right incisive bone
5 Stratum cavernosum of the hard palate (palatine venous plexus)
6 Minor labial salivary glands

7 Intrinsic muscles of the tongue (apex)
8 Reserve crown of tooth 301 (left inferior central incisor)
9 Reserve crown of tooth 302 (left inferior intermediate incisor)
10 Reserve crown of tooth 303 (left inferior corner incisor)

11 Palatine process of incisive bone
12 Palatine fissure
13 Orbicularis oris m.
14 Greater palatine a.
15 Nasal venous plexus
16 Inferior (mandibular) incisive m.
17 Vomeronasal duct

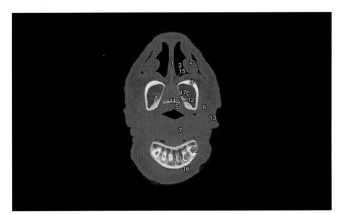

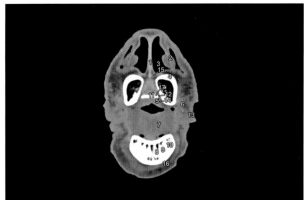

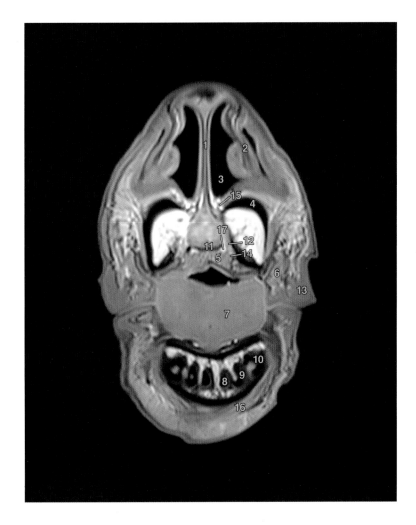

T6

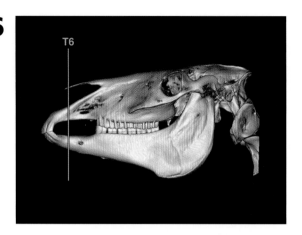

1. Bones of the head
2. Oral and dental structures
3. Nasal and sinus structures
4. Larynx, pharynx, and guttural pouches
5. Ophthalmic structures
6. Auricular structures
7. Brain and nervous system
8. Vascular anatomy
9. Muscles
10. Glandular structures – lymph and salivary

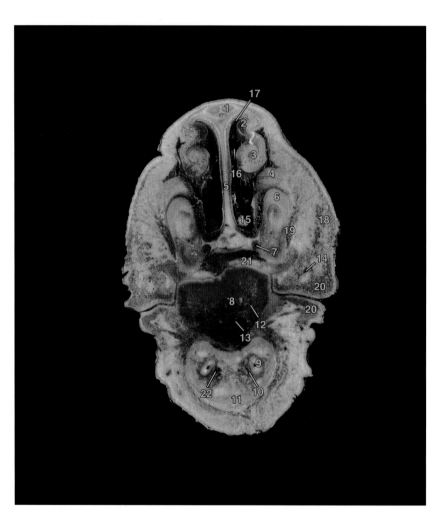

1 Rostral extent nasal bone
2 Straight fold of the dorsal conchae
3 Alar fold of the dorsal conchae (medial accessory nasal cartilage)
4 Basal fold of the ventral conchae
5 Nasal septum
6 Nasal process of the incisive bone
7 Vomeronasal organ
8 Intrinsic muscles of the tongue

9 Reserve crown of tooth 303 (left inferior corner incisor)
10 Dental branch of the inferior alveolar a.
11 Mandible
12 Lingual v.
13 Deep lingual a.
14 Labialis superior v.
15 Ventral nasal meatus
16 Common nasal meatus

17 Dorsal nasal meatus
18 Levator nasolabialis m.
19 Caninus m.
20 Orbicularis oris m.
21 Body of the incisive bone (rostral hard palate)
22 Dental branch of the inferior alveolar v.

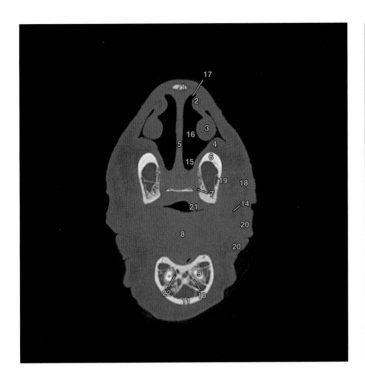

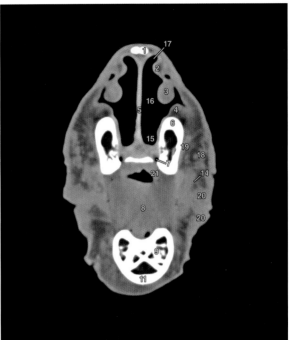

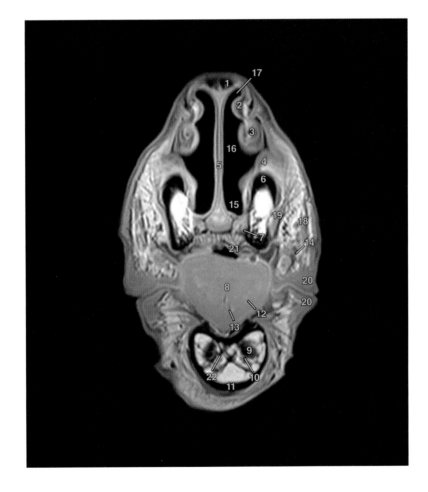

T7

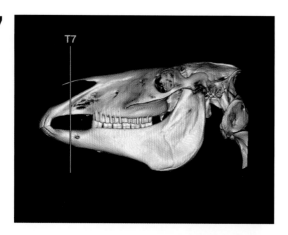

1. **Bones of the head**
2. **Oral and dental structures**
3. **Nasal and sinus structures**
4. Larynx, pharynx, and guttural pouches
5. **Ophthalmic structures**
6. **Auricular structures**
7. Brain and nervous system
8. **Vascular anatomy**
9. Muscles
10. **Glandular structures – lymph and salivary**

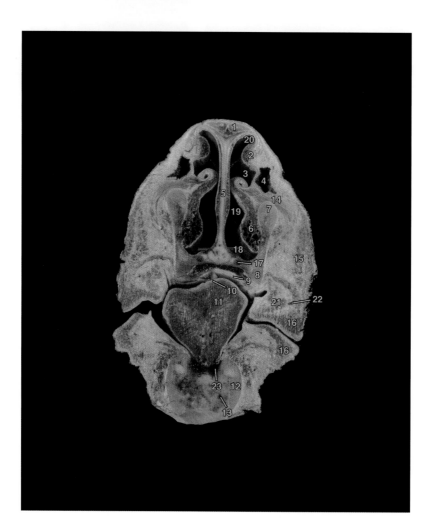

1 Nasal bone	9 Mucosa of the hard palate	17 Vomeronasal organ
2 Dorsal concha	10 Tunica mucosa of the tongue	18 Ventral nasal meatus
3 Middle meatus	11 Intrinsic muscles of the tongue	19 Common nasal meatus
4 Nasal diverticulum	12 Mandible	20 Dorsal nasal meatus
5 Nasal septum	13 Mandibular canal	21 Minor labial salivary glands
6 Ventral concha	14 Dorsal part of lateral nasal m.	22 Labialis superior v.
7 Nasal process of incisive bone	15 Levator nasolabialis m.	23 Sublingual a. and v.
8 Maxilla	16 Orbicularis oris m.	

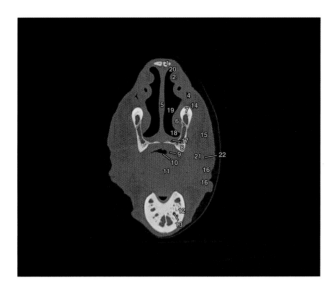

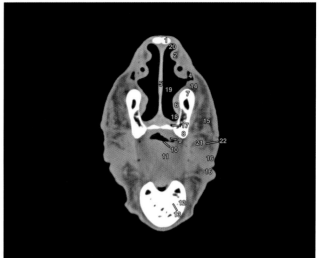

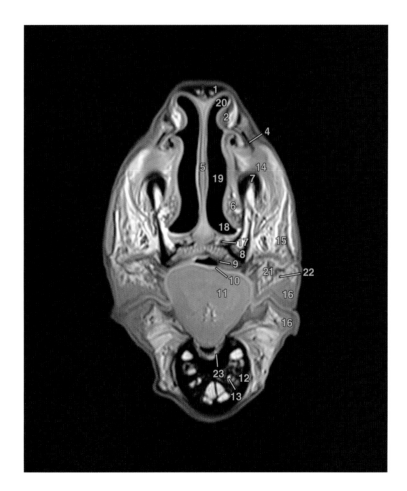

T8

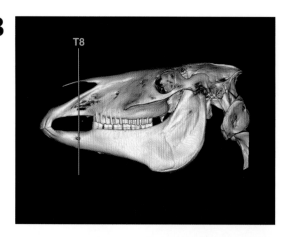

1. **Bones of the head**
2. **Oral and dental structures**
3. **Nasal and sinus structures**
4. Larynx, pharynx, and guttural pouches
5. **Ophthalmic structures**
6. **Auricular structures**
7. Brain and nervous system
8. **Vascular anatomy**
9. Muscles
10. **Glandular structures – lymph and salivary**

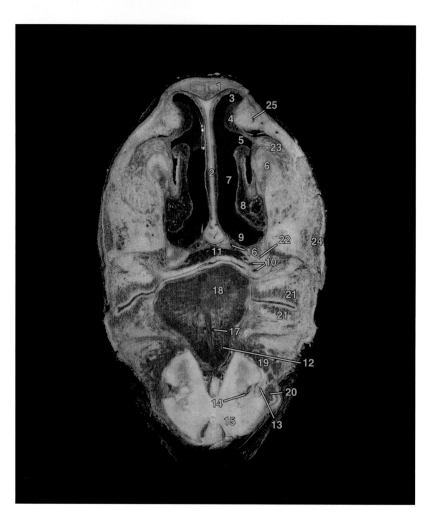

1 Nasal bone	10 Major palatine a. and v.	19 Buccinator m.
2 Nasal septum	11 Stratum cavernosum of the hard palate	20 Depressor labii inferioris m.
3 Dorsal meatus	12 Genioglossus m.	21 Orbicularis oris m.
4 Dorsal concha	13 Mental foramen	**22 maxilla**
5 Middle meatus	14 Mandibular canal	23 Dorsal part of lateral nasal m.
6 Incisive bone	15 Mandible	24 Caninus m.
7 Common meatus	16 Vomeronasal organ	25 Levator labii superioris m.
8 Ventral concha	17 Deep lingual v.	
9 Ventral meatus	18 Intrinsic muscle of tongue	

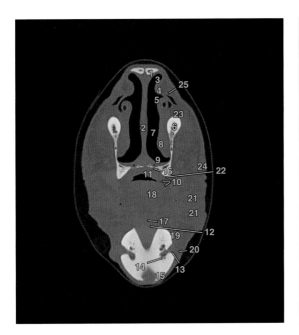

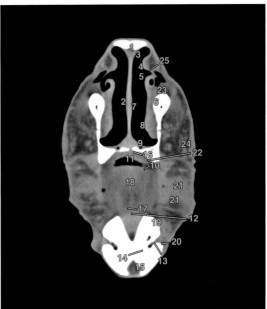

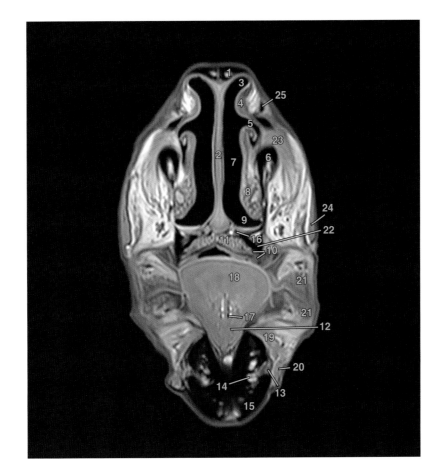

T9

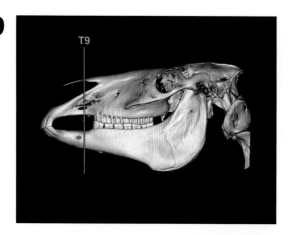

1. **Bones of the head**
2. Oral and dental structures
3. **Nasal and sinus structures**
4. Larynx, pharynx, and guttural pouches
5. Ophthalmic structures
6. Auricular structures
7. Brain and nervous system
8. **Vascular anatomy**
9. Muscles
10. Glandular structures – lymph and salivary

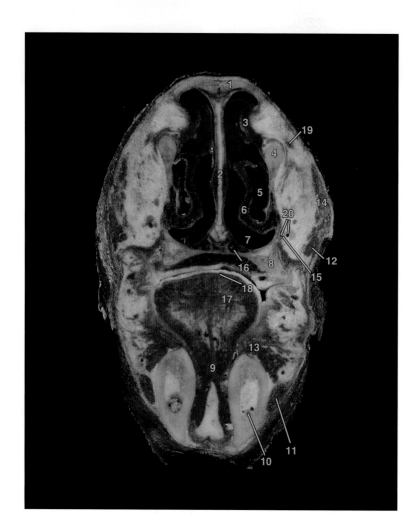

1 Nasal bone	8 Maxilla	15 Branch of infraorbital n.
2 Nasal septum	9 Genioglossus m.	16 Vomeronasal organ
3 Dorsal concha	10 Mandibular canal with inferior alveolar n.	17 Intrinsic muscle of tongue
4 Incisive bone	11 Depressor labii inferioris m.	18 Lingual aponeurosis
5 Ventral conchal bulla	12 Caninus m.	19 Levator labii superioris m.
6 Ventral concha	13 Buccinator m.	20 Lateral nasal a. and v.
7 Ventral meatus	14 Levator nasolabialis m.	

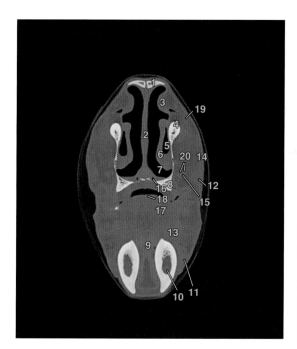

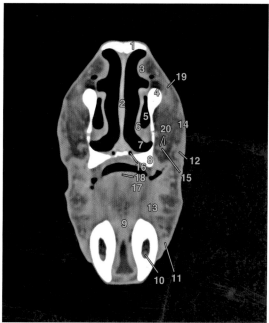

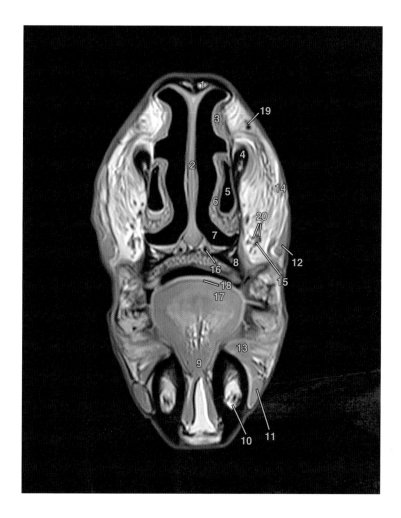

T10

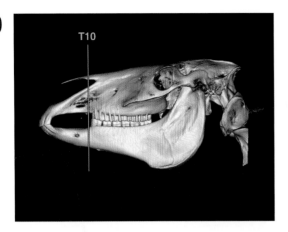

1. **Bones of the head**
2. **Oral and dental structures**
3. **Nasal and sinus structures**
4. Larynx, pharynx, and guttural pouches
5. **Ophthalmic structures**
6. **Auricular structures**
7. Brain and nervous system
8. **Vascular anatomy**
9. Muscles
10. **Glandular structures – lymph and salivary**

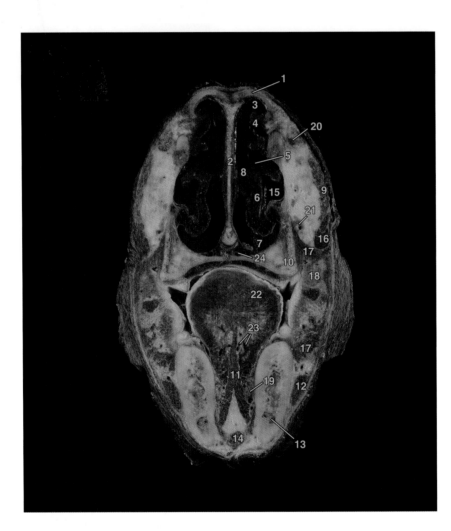

1 Nasal bone	9 Levator nasolabialis m.	17 Buccinator m.
2 Nasal septum	**10 Maxilla**	**18 Ventral buccal salivary gland**
3 Dorsal meatus	11 Genioglossus m.	**19 Polystomatic sublingual salivary gland**
4 Dorsal concha	12 Depressor labii inferioris m.	20 Levator labii superioris m.
5 Middle meatus	**13 Mandibular canal with inferior alveolar n.**	21 Branch of infraorbital n.
6 Ventral concha	14 Geniohyoideus m.	**22 Intrinsic muscles of tongue**
7 Ventral meatus	**15 Ventral conchal bulla**	**23 Deep lingual a. and v.**
8 Common meatus	16 Caninus m.	**24 Vomeronasal organ**

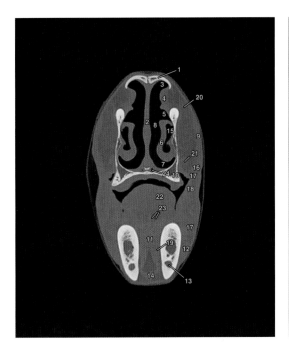

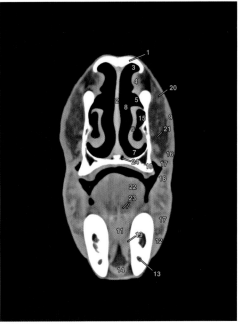

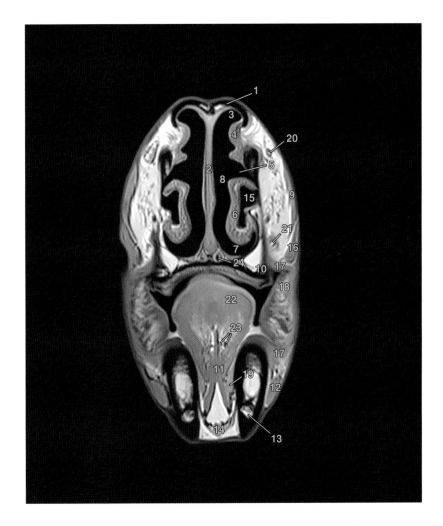

T11

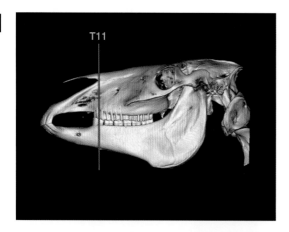

1. **Bones of the head**
2. Oral and dental structures
3. **Nasal and sinus structures**
4. Larynx, pharynx, and guttural pouches
5. **Ophthalmic structures**
6. **Auricular structures**
7. Brain and nervous system
8. **Vascular anatomy**
9. Muscles
10. **Glandular structures – lymph and salivary**

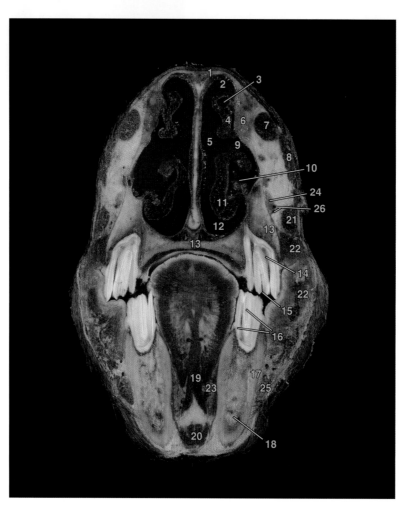

1 **Nasal bone**
2 **Dorsal nasal meatus**
3 **Dorsal conchal bulla**
4 **Dorsal concha**
5 **Common meatus**
6 **Incisive bone**
7 Levator labii superioris m.
8 Levator nasolabialis m.
9 **Middle meatus**
10 **Ventral conchal bulla**

11 **Ventral concha**
12 **Ventral meatus**
13 **Maxilla**
14 Cavum dentis (pulp chamber) tooth 206 (left superior second premolar)
15 Infundibulum, tooth 206 (left superior second premolar)
16 Enamel, tooth 306 (left inferior second premolar)
17 **Mandibular cortex**

18 Mandibular canal (artery, vein, nerve)
19 Genioglossus m.
20 Geniohyoideus m.
21 Caninus m.
22 Buccinator m.
23 **Polystomatic sublingual salivary gland**
24 Infraorbital n.
25 Depressor labii inferioris m.
26 **Lateral nasal a. and v.**

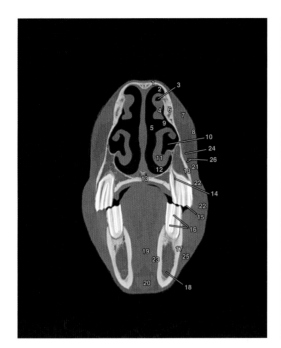

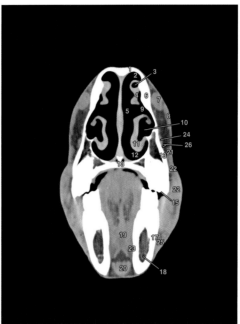

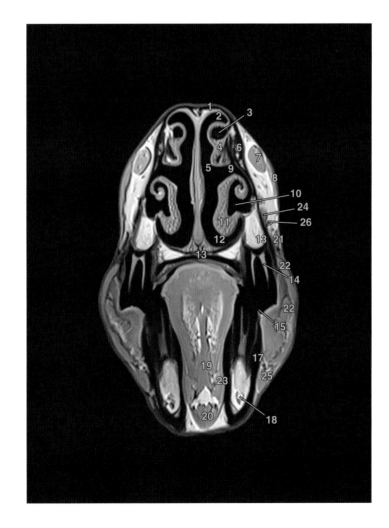

T12

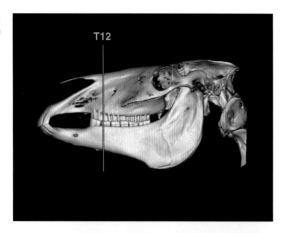

1. **Bones of the head**
2. Oral and dental structures
3. **Nasal and sinus structures**
4. Larynx, pharynx, and guttural pouches
5. **Ophthalmic structures**
6. **Auricular structures**
7. Brain and nervous system
8. **Vascular anatomy**
9. Muscles
10. **Glandular structures – lymph and salivary**

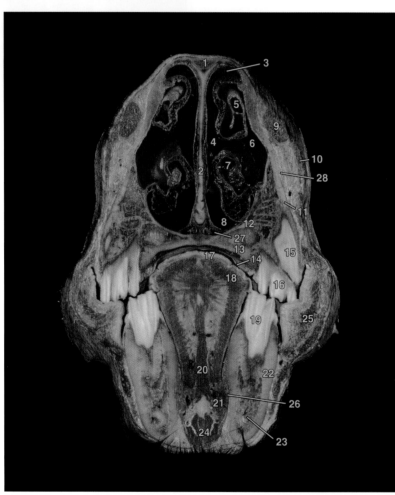

1 Nasal bone	12 Maxilla – nasal surface	20 Genioglossus m.
2 Nasal septum	13 Maxilla – palatine surface	21 Polystomatic sublingual salivary gland
3 Dorsal nasal meatus	14 Mucosa of the hard palate	22 Mandibular cortex
4 Common nasal meatus	15 Reserve crown of tooth 207 (left superior third premolar)	23 Mandibular canal with inferior alveolar a., v., and n.
5 Dorsal conchal bulla	16 Reserve crown of tooth 206 (left superior second premolar)	24 Geniohyoideus m.
6 Middle nasal meatus	17 Tunica mucosa of the tongue	25 Buccinator m.
7 Ventral conchal bulla	18 Intrinsic muscles of the tongue	26 Mylohyoideus m.
8 Ventral nasal meatus	19 Crown of tooth 306 (left inferior second premolar)	27 Vomeronasal organ
9 Levator labii superioris m.		28 Infraorbital n.
10 Levator nasolabialis m.		
11 Maxilla – facial surface		

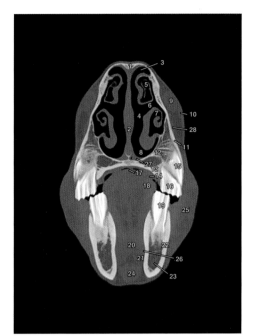

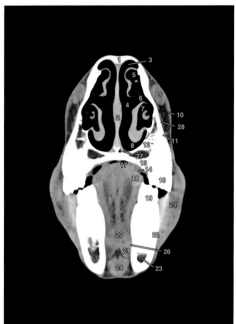

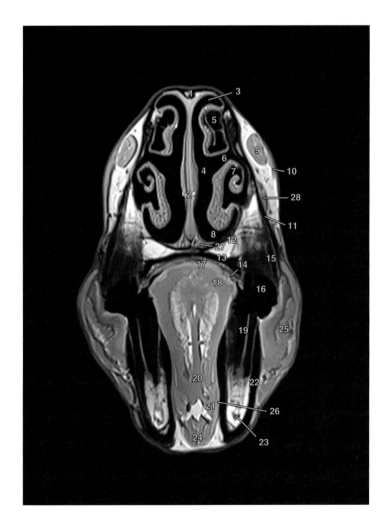

T13

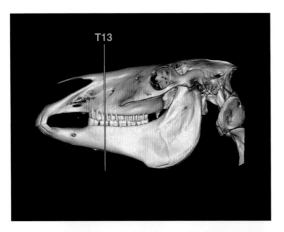

1. **Bones of the head**
2. **Oral and dental structures**
3. **Nasal and sinus structures**
4. Larynx, pharynx, and guttural pouches
5. **Ophthalmic structures**
6. **Auricular structures**
7. Brain and nervous system
8. **Vascular anatomy**
9. Muscles
10. **Glandular structures – lymph and salivary**

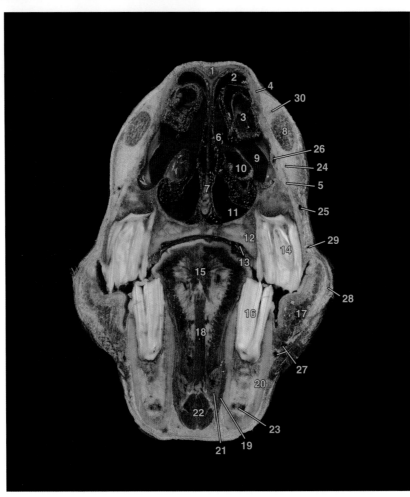

1 Nasal bone	12 Maxilla – palatine surface	23 Mandibular canal with inferior alveolar
2 Dorsal nasal meatus	13 Major palatine a. and v.	a., v., and n.
3 Dorsal conchal bulla	14 Tooth 207 (left superior third premolar)	24 Infraorbital n.
4 Maxilla	15 Intrinsic muscles of the tongue	25 Lateral nasal a. and v.
5 Maxilla – facial surface	16 Tooth 307 (left inferior third premolar)	26 Rostral maxillary alveolar branch of
6 Common nasal meatus	17 Buccinator m.	infraorbital n.
7 Nasal septum	18 Genioglossus m.	27 Inferior labial a. and v.
8 Levator labii superioris m.	19 Mylohyoideus m.	28 Cutaneous facial m.
9 Middle nasal meatus	20 Body of the mandible	29 Superior labial a.
10 Ventral conchal bulla	21 Polystomatic sublingual salivary gland	30 Dorsal nasal a. and v.
11 Ventral nasal meatus	22 Geniohyoideus m.	

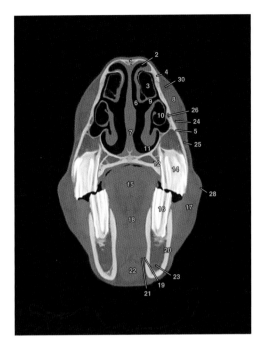

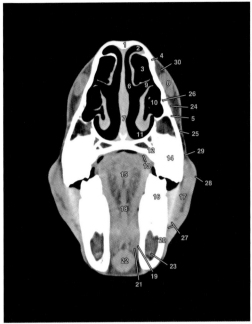

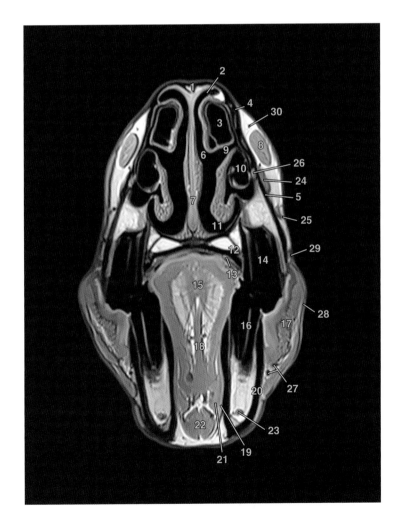

T14

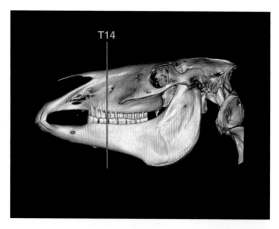

1. **Bones of the head**
2. Oral and dental structures
3. **Nasal and sinus structures**
4. Larynx, pharynx, and guttural pouches
5. **Ophthalmic structures**
6. **Auricular structures**
7. Brain and nervous system
8. **Vascular anatomy**
9. Muscles
10. **Glandular structures – lymph and salivary**

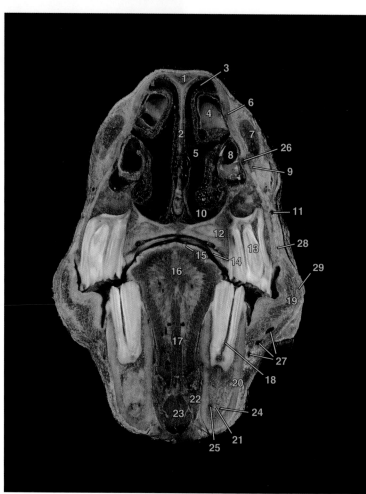

1 Nasal bone	12 Maxilla	22 Polystomatic sublingual salivary gland
2 Nasal septum	13 Tooth 207 (left superior third premolar)	23 Geniohyoideus m.
3 Dorsal nasal meatus	14 Mucosa of the hard palate	24 Inferior alveolar v.
4 Dorsal conchal bulla	15 Tunica mucosa lingua	25 Inferior alveolar a.
5 Common nasal meatus	16 Intrinsic muscles of the tongue	26 Rostral maxillary alveolar branch of
6 Maxilla – facial surface	17 Genioglossus m.	infraorbital n.
7 Levator labii superioris m.	18 Cavum dentis (pulp chamber) tooth 307	27 Inferior labial a. and vv.
8 Ventral conchal bulla	(left inferior third premolar)	28 Superior labial a.
9 Infraorbital n.	19 Buccinator m.	29 Cutaneous facial m.
10 Ventral nasal meatus	20 Mandibular cortex	
11 Lateral nasal a. and v.	21 Inferior alveolar n.	

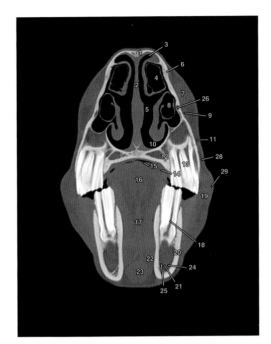

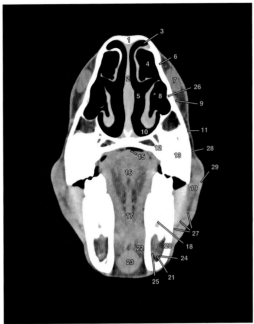

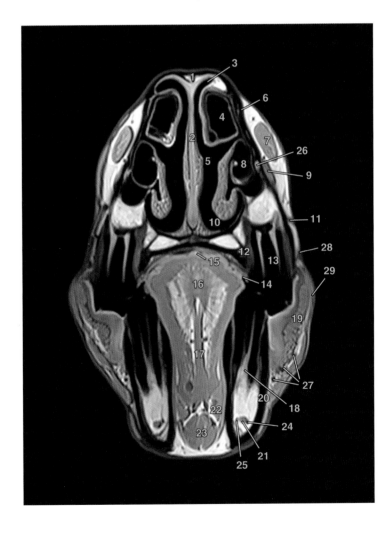

T15

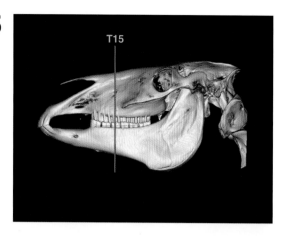

1. **Bones of the head**
2. **Oral and dental structures**
3. **Nasal and sinus structures**
4. Larynx, pharynx, and guttural pouches
5. **Ophthalmic structures**
6. **Auricular structures**
7. Brain and nervous system
8. **Vascular anatomy**
9. Muscles
10. **Glandular structures – lymph and salivary**

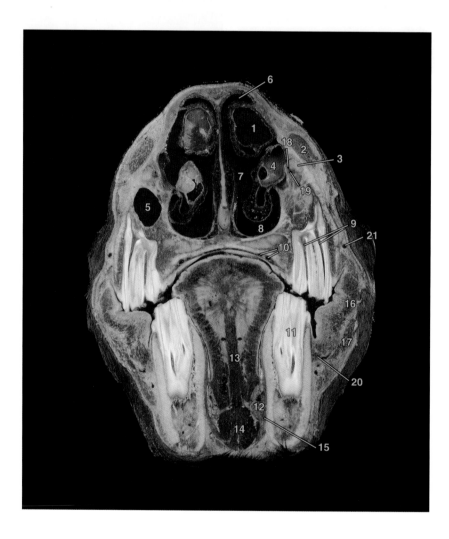

1 Dorsal conchal bulla	**9** Cavum dentis (pulp chambers) tooth 208	16 Buccinator m. (molar part)
2 Levator labii superioris m.	(left superior fourth premolar)	17 Buccinator m. (buccal part)
3 Infraorbital n. (in infraorbital canal)	**10** Major palatine a. and v.	**18** Infraorbital a.
4 Ventral conchal bulla	**11** Tooth 308 (left inferior fourth premolar)	**19** Infraorbital v.
5 Rostral maxillary sinus	**12** Polystomatic sublingual salivary gland	**20** Minor buccal salivary gland
6 Dorsal meatus	13 Genioglossus m.	**21** Superior labial a. and v.
7 Common meatus	14 Geniohyoideus m.	
8 Ventral meatus	15 Mylohyoideus m.	

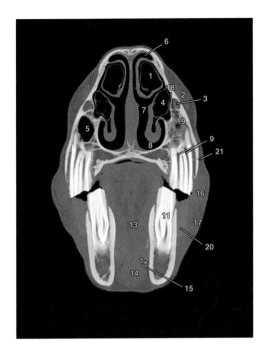

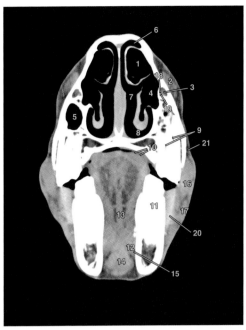

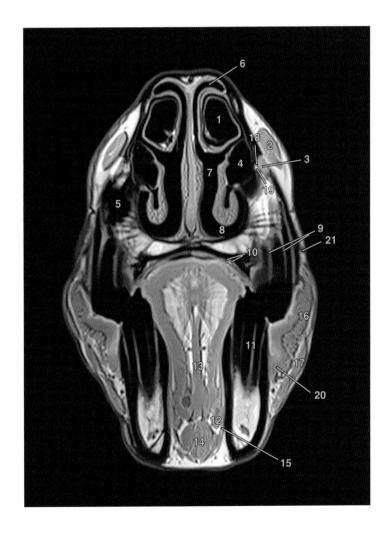

T16

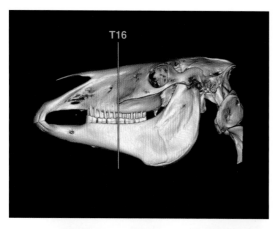

1. Bones of the head
2. Oral and dental structures
3. Nasal and sinus structures
4. Larynx, pharynx, and guttural pouches
5. Ophthalmic structures
6. Auricular structures
7. Brain and nervous system
8. Vascular anatomy
9. Muscles
10. Glandular structures – lymph and salivary

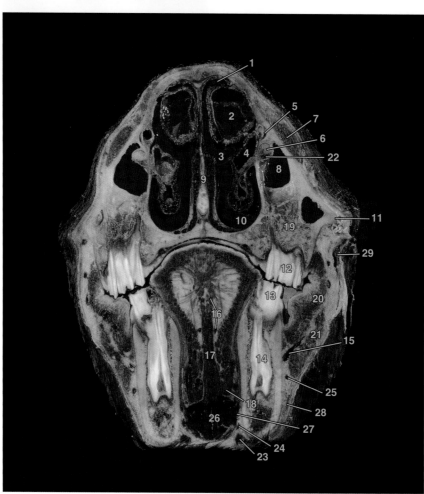

1 Dorsal nasal meatus
2 Dorsal conchal bulla
3 Common nasal meatus
4 Ventral conchal bulla
5 Nasolacrimal duct
6 Infraorbital n.
7 Levator labii superioris m.
8 Rostral maxillary sinus
9 Nasal septum
10 Ventral nasal meatus
11 Facial crest

12 Tooth 209 (left superior first molar)
13 Tooth 309 (left inferior first molar)
   (exposed crown)
14 Tooth 308 (left inferior fourth premolar)
   (reserve crown)
15 Facial v.
16 Lingual a. and v.
17 Genioglossus m.
18 Hyoglossal m.
19 Body of maxilla
20 Buccinator m. (molar part)

21 Buccinator m. (buccal part)
22 Infraorbital a. and v.
23 Digastricus m. (rostral belly)
24 Sublingual a. and v.
25 Inferior labial a.
26 Geniohyoideus m.
27 Mylohyoideus m.
28 Cutaneous facial m.
29 Zygomaticus m.

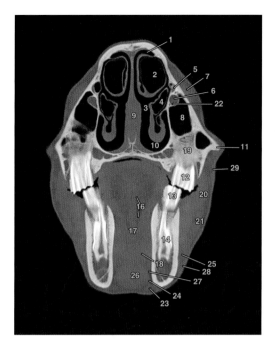

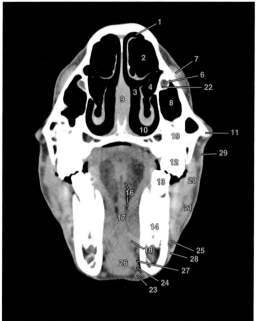

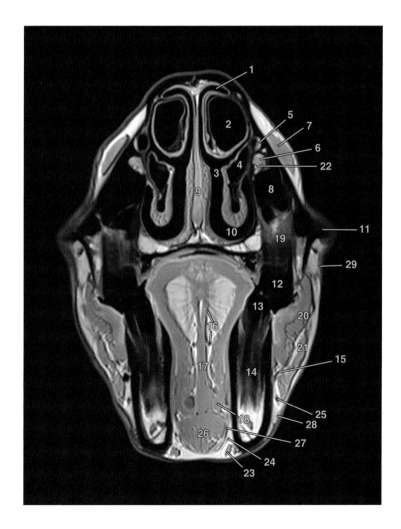

T17

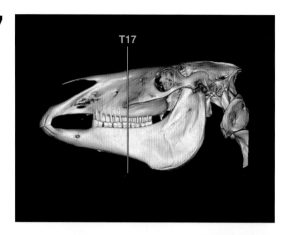

1. **Bones of the head**
2. Oral and dental structures
3. **Nasal and sinus structures**
4. Larynx, pharynx, and guttural pouches
5. Ophthalmic structures
6. Auricular structures
7. Brain and nervous system
8. **Vascular anatomy**
9. Muscles
10. **Glandular structures – lymph and salivary**

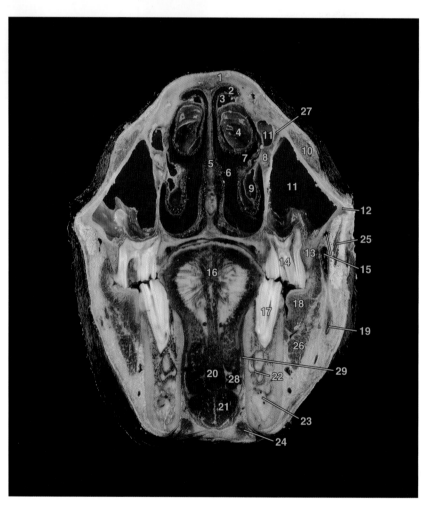

1 Nasal bone	**11 Rostral maxillary sinus**	21 Geniohyoideus m.
2 Dorsal nasal meatus	**12 Facial crest**	**22 Root of tooth 208 (left inferior fourth premolar)**
3 Dorsal conchal sinus (rostral extent)	**13 Maxilla**	23 Inferior alveolar n. in mandibular canal
4 Dorsal conchal bulla	**14 Tooth 209 (left superior first molar)**	24 Digastricus m. (rostral belly)
5 Nasal septum	**15 Deep facial v.**	25 Masseter m.
6 Common nasal meatus	16 Intrinsic muscles of the tongue	26 Buccinator m. (buccal part)
7 Middle nasal meatus	17 Tooth 309 (left inferior first molar)	**27 Nasolacrimal duct**
8 Infraorbital n.	18 Buccinator m. (molar part)	28 Hyoglossus m.
9 Ventral conchal bulla	**19 Facial v.**	29 Mylohyoideus m.
10 Levator labii superioris m.	20 Genioglossus m.	

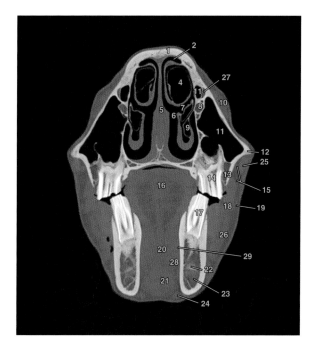

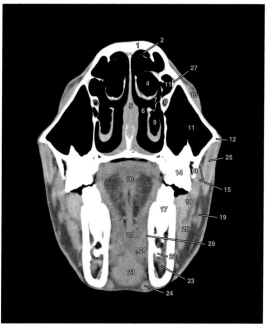

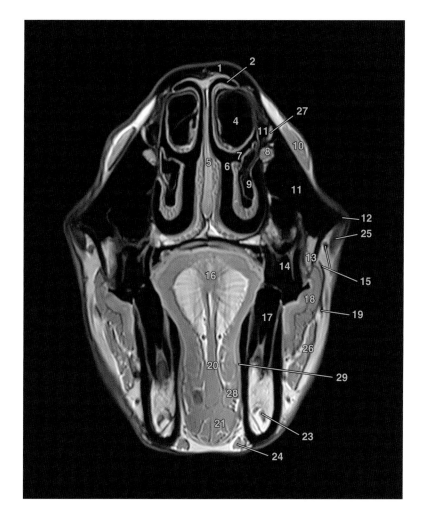

T18

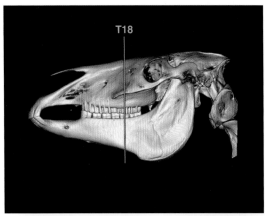

1. **Bones of the head**
2. **Oral and dental structures**
3. **Nasal and sinus structures**
4. Levator labii superioris m. / Larynx, pharynx, and guttural pouches
5. **Ophthalmic structures**
6. **Auricular structures**
7. Brain and nervous system
8. **Vascular anatomy**
9. Muscles
10. **Glandular structures – lymph and salivary**

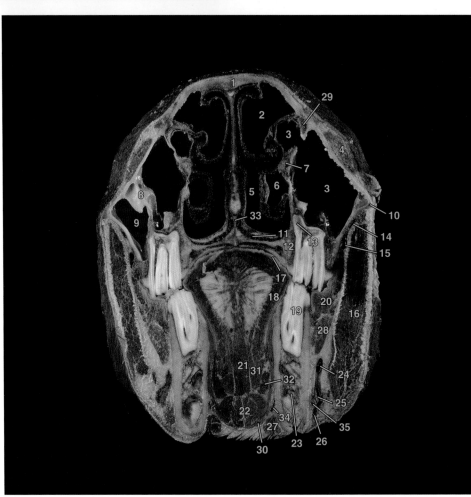

1 Nasal bone	**12 Palantine process of the maxilla and**
2 Conchofrontal sinus	**palatine a.**
3 Rostral maxillary sinus	**13 Mesiolingual (mesiopalatal) root of tooth**
4 Levator labii superioris m.	**210 (left superior second molar)**
5 Common nasal meatus	**14 Transverse facial v.**
6 Ventral conchal sinus	**15 Deep facial v.**
7 Infraorbital a., v., and n.	16 Masseter m.
8 Septum between rostral and caudal	17 Lingual mucosa
maxillary sinuses	18 Intrinsic muscles of the tongue
9 Caudal maxillary sinus	19 Tooth 310 (left inferior second molar)
10 Facial crest	20 Buccinator m. (molar part)
11 Nasal submucosa, venous	21 Genioglossus m.
plexus	22 Geniohyoideus m.

23 Inferior alveolar n. in mandibular canal	
24 Buccal v.	
25 Facial v.	
26 Facial a.	
27 Digastricus m. (rostral belly)	
28 Buccinator m. (buccal part)	
29 Nasolacrimal duct	
30 Mylohyoideus m.	
31 Hyoglossus m.	
32 Styloglossus m.	
33 Vomer	
34 Sublingual a. and v.	
35 Parotid duct	

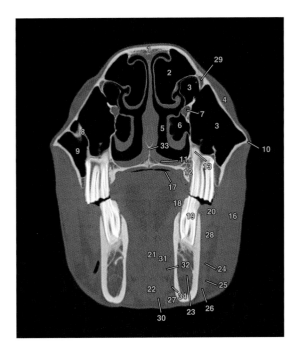

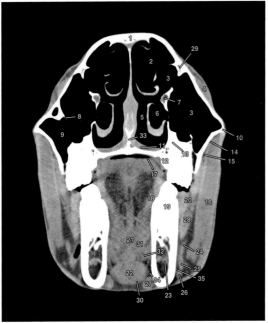

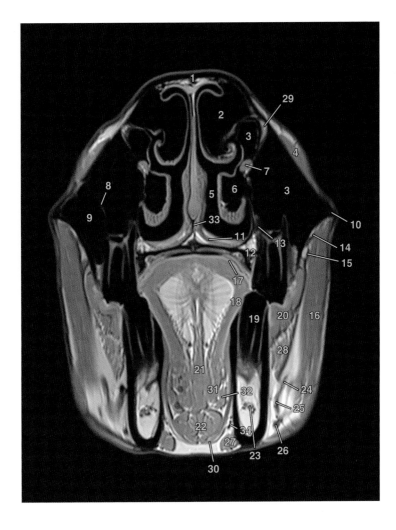

T19

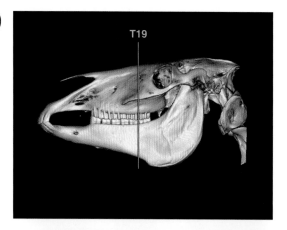

1. **Bones of the head**
2. Oral and dental structures
3. **Nasal and sinus structures**
4. Larynx, pharynx, and guttural pouches
5. **Ophthalmic structures**
6. **Auricular structures**
7. Brain and nervous system
8. **Vascular anatomy**
9. Muscles
10. **Glandular structures – lymph and salivary**

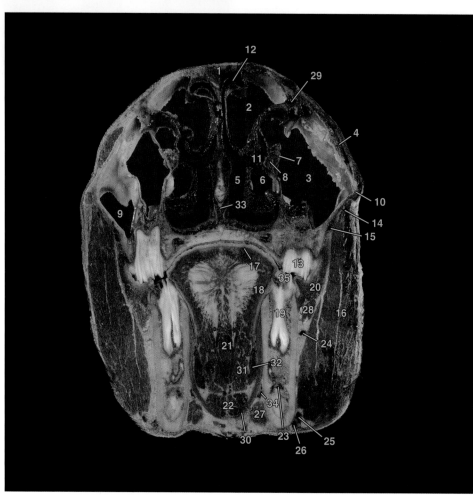

1 Nasal bone	13 Tooth 210 (left superior second molar)	**25 Facial v.**
2 Conchofrontal sinus	**14 Transverse facial v.**	**26 Facial a.**
3 Rostral maxillary sinus	**15 Deep facial v.**	27 Digastricus m. (rostral belly)
4 Levator labii superioris m.	16 Masseter m.	28 Buccinator m. (buccal part)
5 Common nasal meatus	17 Lingual aponeurosis	**29 Nasolacrimal duct**
6 Ventral conchal sinus	18 Intrinsic muscles of the tongue	30 Mylohyoideus m.
7 Infraorbital canal	19 Tooth 310 (left inferior second molar)	31 Hyoglossus m.
8 Infraorbital n.	20 Buccinator m. (molar part)	32 Styloglossus m.
9 Caudal maxillary sinus	21 Genioglossus m.	**33 Vomer**
10 Facial crest	22 Geniohyoideus m.	**34 Sublingual a. and v.**
11 Middle nasal meatus	23 Inferior alveolar n. in mandibular canal	**35 Tooth 311 (left inferior third molar)**
12 Dorsal nasal meatus	**24 Buccal v.**	

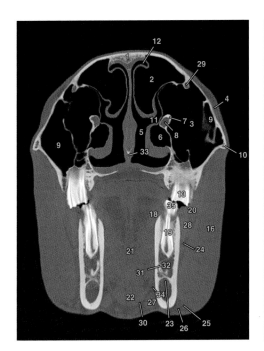

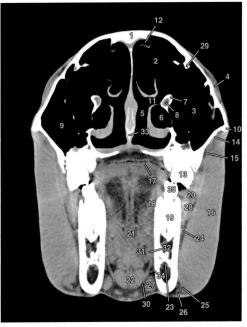

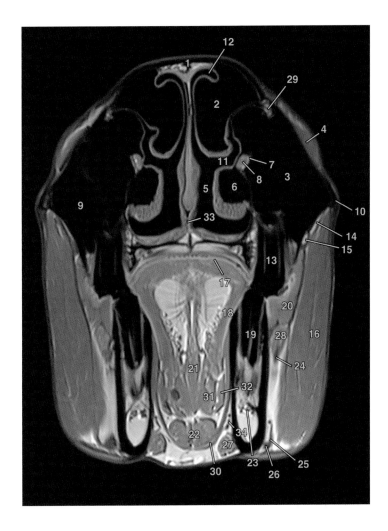

T20

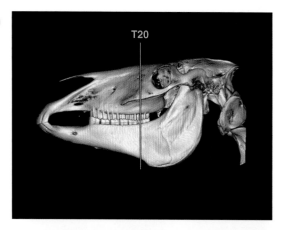

1. **Bones of the head**
2. Oral and dental structures
3. **Nasal and sinus structures**
4. Larynx, pharynx, and guttural pouches
5. **Ophthalmic structures**
6. **Auricular structures**
7. Brain and nervous system
8. **Vascular anatomy**
9. Muscles
10. **Glandular structures – lymph and salivary**

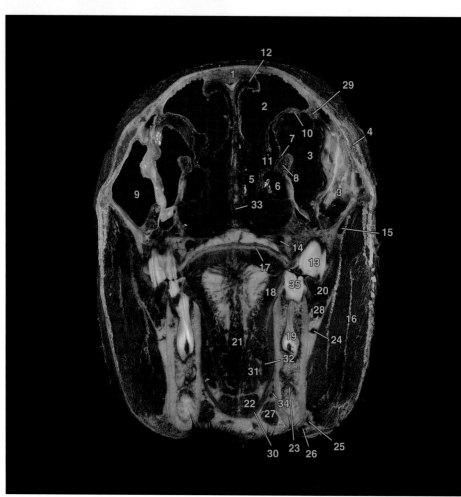

1 Nasal bone	**13 Tooth 211 (left superior third molar)**	**25 Facial v.**
2 Conchofrontal sinus	**14 Major palatine a. and v.**	**26 Facial a.**
3 Rostral maxillary sinus	**15 Deep facial v.**	27 Digastricus m. (rostral belly)
4 Levator labii superioris m.	16 Masseter m.	28 Buccinator m. (buccal part)
5 Common nasal meatus	**17 Lingual mucosa**	**29 Nasolacrimal duct**
6 Ventral conchal sinus	**18 Intrinsic muscles of the tongue**	30 Mylohyoideus m.
7 Conchomaxillary opening	**19 Tooth 310 (left inferior second molar)**	31 Hyoglossus m.
8 Infraorbital n.	20 Buccinator m. (molar part)	32 Styloglossus m.
9 Caudal maxillary sinus	21 Genioglossus m.	**33 Vomer**
10 Nasomaxillary opening	22 Geniohyoideus m.	**34 Sublingual a. and v.**
11 Middle nasal meatus	23 Inferior alveolar n. in mandibular canal	**35 Tooth 311 (left inferior third molar)**
12 Dorsal nasal meatus	24 Buccal a., v. and n.	

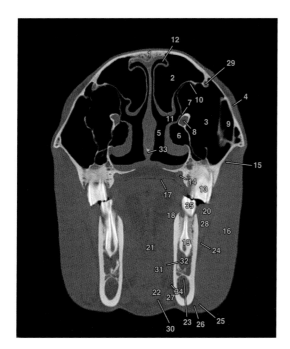

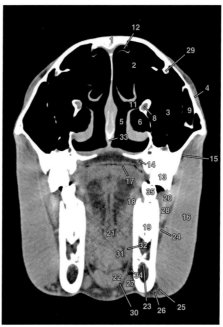

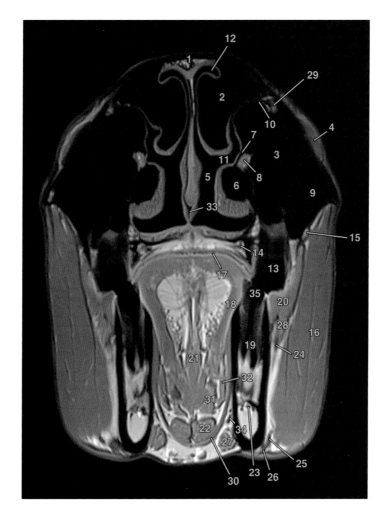

T21

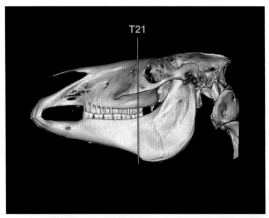

1. **Bones of the head**
2. **Oral and dental structures**
3. **Nasal and sinus structures**
4. Larynx, pharynx, and guttural pouches
5. **Ophthalmic structures**
6. **Auricular structures**
7. Brain and nervous system
8. **Vascular anatomy**
9. Muscles
10. **Glandular structures – lymph and salivary**

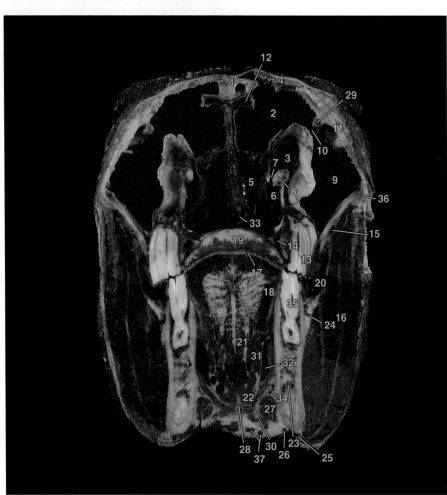

1 Frontal bone	14 Major palatine a. and v.	27 Digastricus m. (rostral belly)
2 Frontal sinus	15 Deep facial v.	28 Lingual process of basihyoid bone
3 Rostral maxillary sinus	16 Masseter m.	29 Nasolacrimal duct
4 Nasal bone	17 Lingual mucosa	30 Mylohyoideus m.
5 Common nasal meatus	18 Intrinsic muscles of the tongue	31 Hyoglossus m.
6 Ventral conchal sinus	19 Soft palate	32 Styloglossus m.
7 Conchomaxillary opening	20 Buccinator m. (molar part)	33 Vomer
8 Infraorbital n.	21 Genioglossus m.	34 Sublingual a. and v.
9 Caudal maxillary sinus	22 Geniohyoideus m.	35 Tooth 311 (left inferior third molar)
10 Frontomaxillary opening	23 Inferior alveolar n. in mandibular canal	36 Zygomatic bone
11 Lacrimal bone	24 Buccal a., v. and n.	37 Mandibular lymph nodes
12 Dorsal nasal meatus	25 Facial v.	
13 Tooth 211 (left superior third molar)	26 Facial a.	

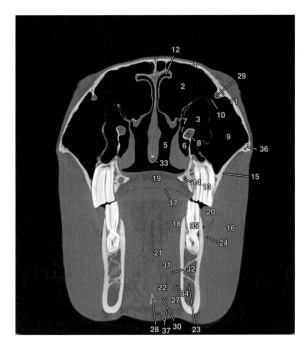

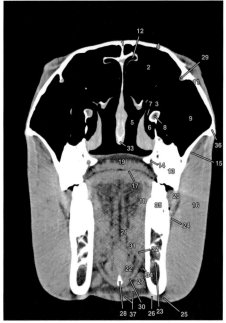

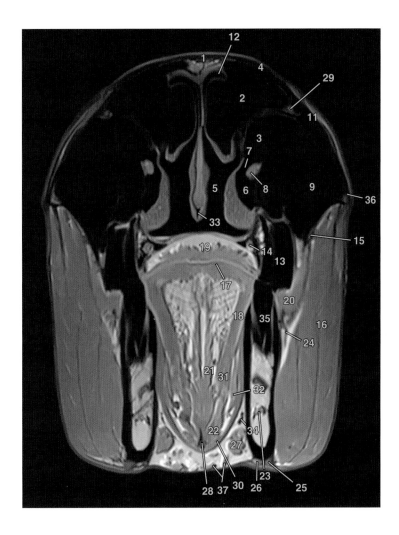

T22

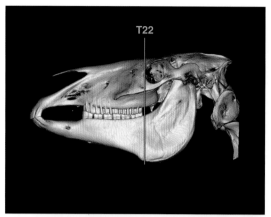

1. **Bones of the head**
2. **Oral and dental structures**
3. **Nasal and sinus structures**
4. Larynx, pharynx, and guttural pouches
5. **Ophthalmic structures**
6. **Auricular structures**
7. Brain and nervous system
8. **Vascular anatomy**
9. Muscles
10. **Glandular structures – lymph and salivary**

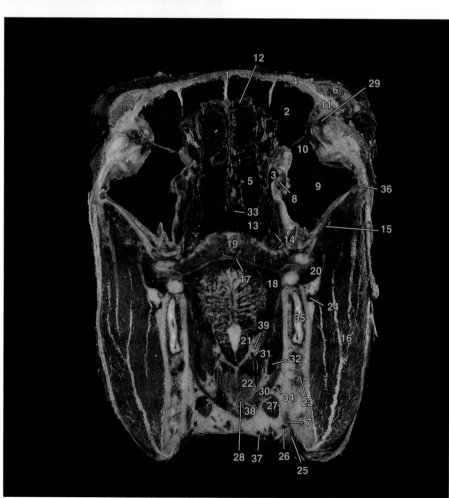

1 Frontal bone	14 Major palatine a. and v.
2 Conchofrontal sinus	15 Deep facial v.
3 Rostral maxillary sinus	16 Masseter m.
4 Nasal bone	17 Lingual mucosa
5 Common nasal meatus	18 Intrinsic muscles of the tongue
6 Orbicularis oculi m.	19 Soft palate
7 Medial pterygoid m. (rostral extent)	20 Buccinator m. (molar part)
8 Infraorbital n.	21 Genioglossus m.
9 Caudal maxillary sinus	22 Geniohyoideus m.
10 Frontomaxillary opening	23 Inferior alveolar n. in mandibular canal
11 Lacrimal bone	24 Buccal a., v. and n.
12 Dorsal nasal meatus	25 Facial v.
13 Left choana	26 Facial a.

27 Digastricus m. (rostral belly)
28 Lingual process of basihyoid bone
29 Nasolacrimal duct
30 Mylohyoideus m.
31 Hyoglossal m.
32 Styloglossal m.
33 Vomer
34 Sublingual a. and v.
35 Tooth 311 (left inferior third molar)
36 Zygomatic bone
37 Mandibular lymph nodes
38 Omohyoideus and sternohyoideus mm.
39 Ceratohyoid bone

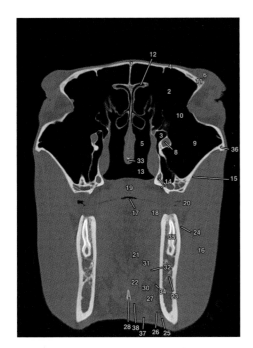
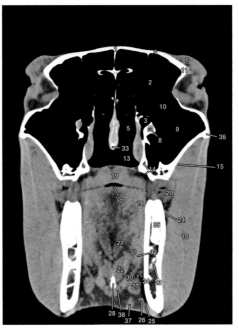
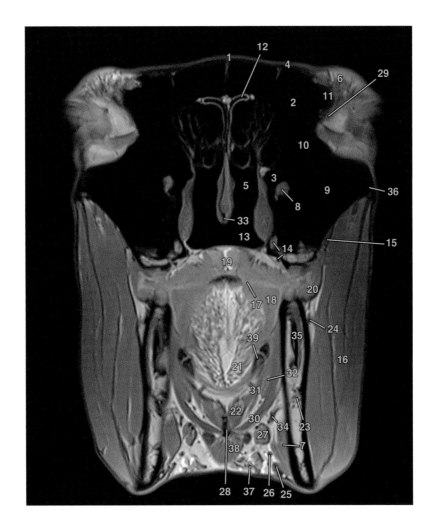

T23

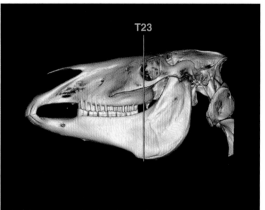

1. **Bones of the head**
2. **Oral and dental structures**
3. **Nasal and sinus structures**
4. Larynx, pharynx, and guttural pouches
5. **Ophthalmic structures**
6. **Auricular structures**
7. Brain and nervous system
8. **Vascular anatomy**
9. Muscles
10. **Glandular structures – lymph and salivary**

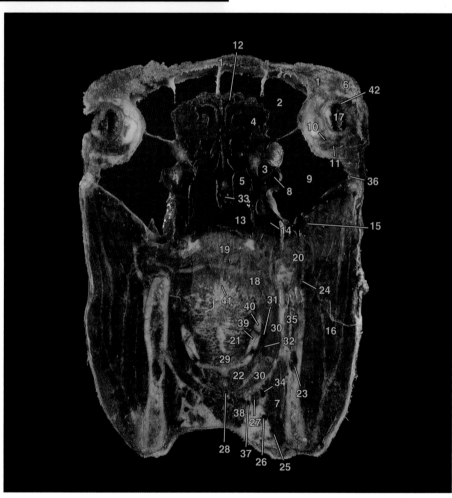

1 Frontal bone	**15 Deep facial v.**	29 Transversus hyoideus m.
2 Conchofrontal sinus	16 Masseter m.	30 Mylohyoideus m.
3 Rostral maxillary sinus	17 Vitreal body	31 Hyoglossus m.
4 Ethmoid turbinates	18 Intrinsic muscles of the tongue	32 Styloglossus m.
5 Common nasal meatus	19 Soft palate	**33 Vomer**
6 Orbicularis oculi m.	20 Buccinator m. (molar part)	**34 Sublingual a. and v.**
7 Medial pterygoid m. (rostral extent)	21 Genioglossus m.	**35 Tooth 311 (left inferior third molar)**
8 Infraorbital n.	22 Geniohyoideus m.	**36 Zygomatic bone**
9 Caudal maxillary sinus	23 Inferior alveolar n. in mandibular canal	**37 Lingual v.**
10 Ventral oblique m.	24 Buccal a., v. and n.	38 Omohyoideus and sternohyoideus mm.
11 Ventral rectus m.	**25 Facial v.**	**39 Ceratohyoid bone**
12 Dorsal nasal meatus	**26 Facial a.**	**40 Stylohyoid bone**
13 Left choana	27 Digastricus m. (rostral belly)	**41 Lingual dorsum cartilage**
14 Major palatine canal	**28 Lingual process of basihyoid bone**	42 Sclera

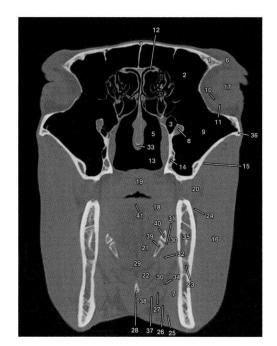

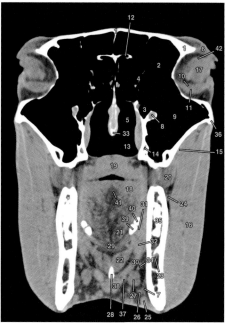

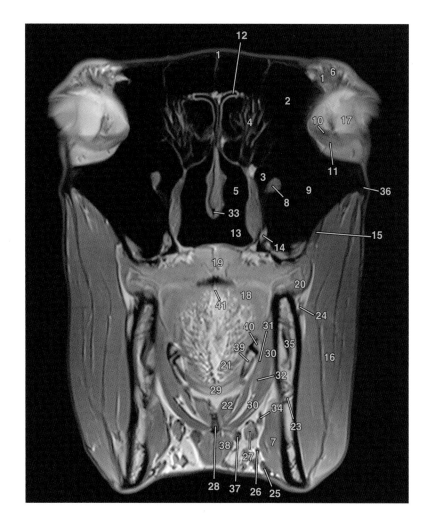

T24

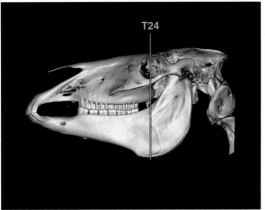

1. **Bones of the head**
2. Oral and dental structures
3. **Nasal and sinus structures**
4. Larynx, pharynx, and guttural pouches
5. Ophthalmic structures
6. **Auricular structures**
7. Brain and nervous system
8. **Vascular anatomy**
9. Muscles
10. **Glandular structures – lymph and salivary**

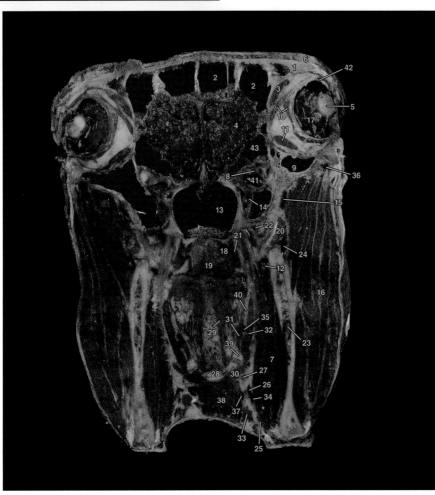

1 Frontal bone	**15 Deep facial v.**	30 Mylohyoideus m.
2 Conchofrontal sinus	16 Masseter m.	31 Ceratohyoideus m.
3 Dorsal rectus m.	**17 Vitreal body**	32 Styloglossus m.
4 Ethmoid turbinates	18 Levator muscle of soft palate	**33 Mandibular lymph node**
5 Lens	19 Tunica mucosa of soft palate	**34 Facial a.**
6 Levator anguli oculi medialis m.	20 Buccinator m. (molar part)	**35 Sublingual a.**
7 Medial pterygoid m.	21 Tensor muscle of soft palate	**36 Transverse facial a. and v.**
8 Infraorbital n.	**22 Major palatine v.**	**37 Sublingual v.**
9 Caudal maxillary sinus	23 Inferior alveolar n. in mandibular canal	38 Omohyoideus and sternohyoideus mm.
10 Retractor bulbi m.	24 Buccal a., v. and n.	**39 Ceratohyoid bone**
11 Ventral rectus m.	**25 Facial v.**	**40 Stylohyoid bone**
12 Dorsal lingual v.	**26 Lingual a.**	**41 Sphenopalatine v.**
13 Left choana	27 Digastricus tendon	42 Sclera
14 Major palatine canal (major palatine a. and n.)	**28 Basihyoid bone**	**43 Sphenopalatinal opening**
	29 Hyoepiglotticus m.	

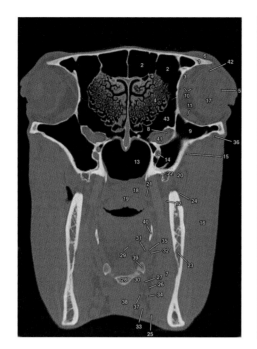

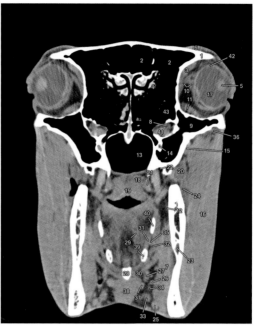

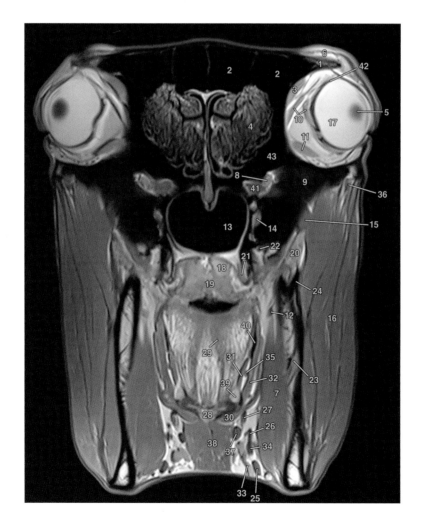

T25

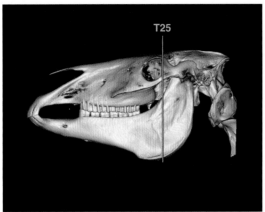

1. **Bones of the head**
2. Oral and dental structures
3. **Nasal and sinus structures**
4. Larynx, pharynx, and guttural pouches
5. **Ophthalmic structures**
6. **Auricular structures**
7. Brain and nervous system
8. **Vascular anatomy**
9. Muscles
10. **Glandular structures – lymph and salivary**

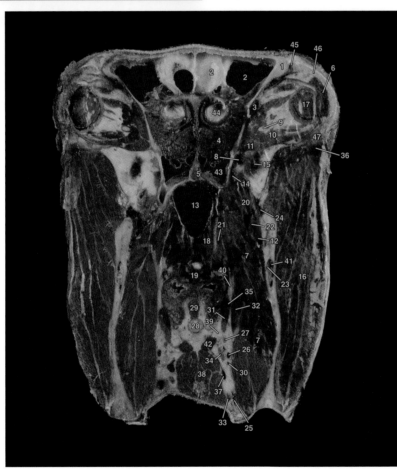

1 Frontal bone	17 Vitreal body	33 Mandibular lymph node
2 Frontal sinus	18 Levator muscle of soft palate	34 Mandibular salivary gland
3 Dorsal rectus m.	19 Soft palate	35 Lingual a.
4 Ethmoid turbinates	20 Lateral pterygoid m.	36 Transverse facial a. and v.
5 Vomer	21 Tensor muscle of soft palate	37 Sublingual v.
6 Lateral rectus m.	22 Maxillary v.	38 Omohyoideus and sternohyoideus mm.
7 Medial pterygoid m.	23 Inferior alveolar n. in mandibular canal	39 Thyrohyoid bone
8 Infraorbital n.	24 Buccal a., v. and n.	40 Stylohyoid bone
9 Optic n.	25 Facial v.	41 Inferior alveolar v.
10 Retractor bulbi m.	26 Facial a.	42 Thyrohyoideus m.
11 Ventral rectus m.	27 Digastricus tendon	43 Sphenopalatinal opening
12 Dorsal lingual v.	28 Epiglottis apex	44 Ethmoidal fossa
13 Nasopharynx	29 Hyoepiglotticus m.	45 Supraorbital foramen and n.
14 Infraorbital a. and major palatine a.	30 Mandibular duct	46 Zygomatic process of frontal bone
15 Deep facial v.	31 Ceratohyoideus m.	47 Zygomatic bone
16 Masseter m.	32 Styloglossus m.	

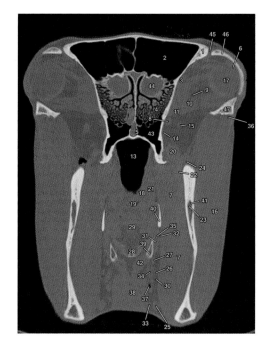

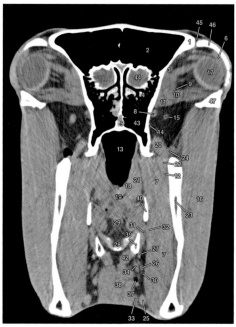

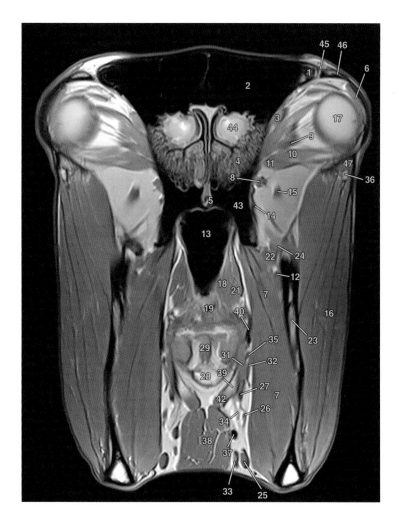

T26

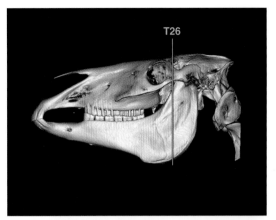

1. **Bones of the head**
2. Oral and dental structures
3. **Nasal and sinus structures**
4. Larynx, pharynx, and guttural pouches
5. Ophthalmic structures
6. **Auricular structures**
7. Brain and nervous system
8. **Vascular anatomy**
9. Muscles
10. **Glandular structures – lymph and salivary**

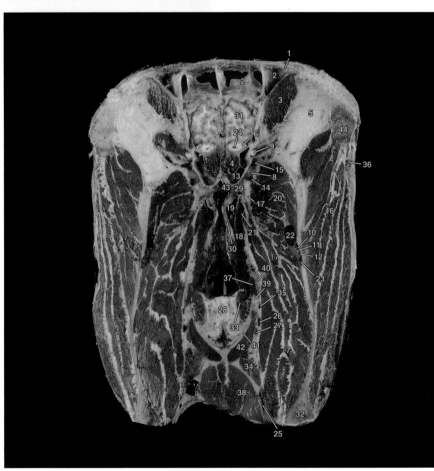

1 Frontal bone	16 Masseter m.	30 Medial lamina of auditory tube
2 Frontal sinus	**17 Pterygoid process of the basisphenoid bone**	31 Cerebral cortex
3 Temporalis m.		**32 Mandible**
4 Ethmoid turbinates (caudal aspect)	18 Levator muscle of soft palate	33 Palatopharyngeus m.
5 Orbital fat body	19 Auditory tube	**34 Mandibular salivary gland**
6 Olfactory lobe	20 Lateral pterygoid m.	**35 Lingual artery**
7 Medial pterygoid m.	21 Tensor muscle of soft palate	**36 Transverse facial a. and v.**
8 Maxillary n.	**22 Maxillary v.**	37 Hyopharyngeus m.
9 Optic n.	**23 Pterygoid branch of maxillary v.**	38 Omohyoideus and sternohyoideus mm.
10 Inferior alveolar a.	24 Rostral horn of lateral ventricle	39 Rostral cornu of thyroid cartilage
11 Inferior alveolar n.	**25 Linguofacial v.**	**40 Stylohyoid bone**
12 Inferior alveolar v.	**26 Facial a.**	41 Thyroid cartilage
13 Sphenopalatine sinus	27 Digastricus tendon	42 Thyrohyoideus m.
14 Infraorbital a. and major palatine a.	**28 Epiglottis**	**43 Vomer**
15 Deep facial v.	**29 Palatine bone**	**44 Zygomatic process of temporal bone**

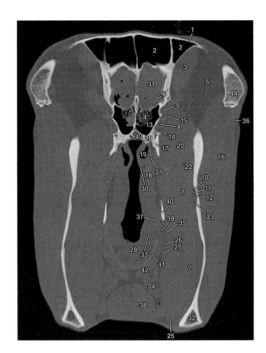

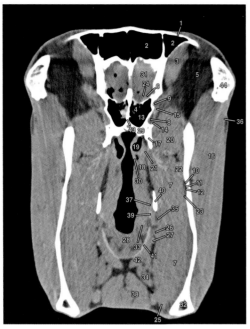

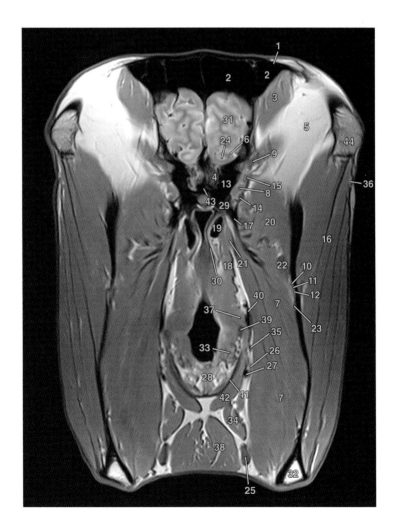

T27

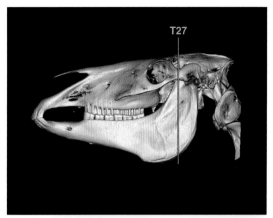

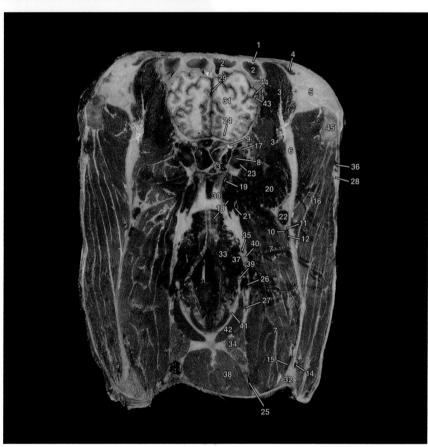

1. **Bones of the head**
2. **Oral and dental structures**
3. **Nasal and sinus structures**
4. Larynx, pharynx, and guttural pouches
5. **Ophthalmic structures**
6. **Auricular structures**
7. Brain and nervous system
8. **Vascular anatomy**
9. Muscles
10. **Glandular structures – lymph and salivary**

1 **Frontal bone**
2 **Frontal sinus**
3 Temporalis m.
4 Frontoscutularis m.
5 **Orbital fat body**
6 **Coronoid process of the mandible**
7 Medial pterygoid m.
8 Maxillary branch of trigeminal n. (in alar canal)
9 Optic n. in optic canal
10 **Inferior alveolar a.**
11 Inferior alveolar n.
12 **Inferior alveolar v.**
13 **Presphenoid bone and sphenopalatine sinus**
14 **Ventral masseteric v. and masseteric branches of external carotid a.**

15 Pterygoid branches of facial a. and v.
16 Masseter m.
17 Oculomotor n., trochlear n., abducens n., and ophthalmic n. (in orbital fissure)
18 Levator muscle of soft palate
19 Auditory tube
20 Lateral pterygoid m.
21 Tensor muscle of soft palate
22 **Maxillary v.**
23 **Maxillary a. (in alar canal)**
24 Rostral horn of lateral ventricle
25 **Linguofacial v.**
26 **Linguofacial trunk**
27 Digastricus tendon
28 Facial n., buccal branch
29 Falx cerebri
30 Medial lamina of auditory tube

31 Cerebral cortex (white matter tracts)
32 **Mandible**
33 Palatopharyngeus m.
34 **Mandibular salivary gland**
35 **Ascending palatine a.**
36 **Transverse facial a. and v.**
37 Hyopharyngeus m.
38 Omohyoideus and sternohyoideus mm.
39 Rostral cornu of thyroid cartilage
40 **Stylohyoid bone**
41 Thyroid cartilage
42 Thyrohyoideus m.
43 Cerebral gyrus
44 Cerebral sulcus
45 **Zygomatic process of temporal bone**

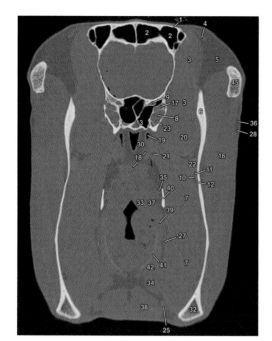
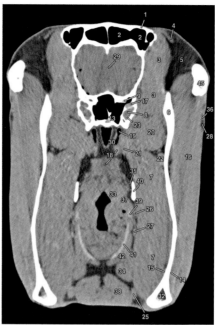
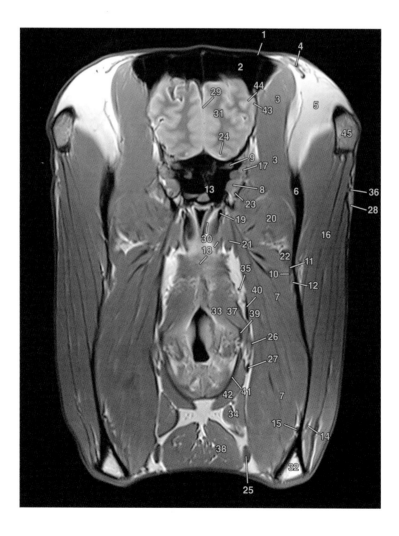

T28

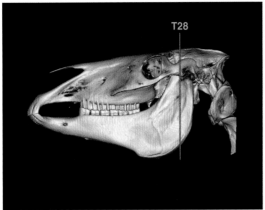

1. Bones of the head
2. Oral and dental structures
3. Nasal and sinus structures
4. Larynx, pharynx, and guttural pouches
5. Ophthalmic structures
6. Auricular structures
7. Brain and nervous system
8. Vascular anatomy
9. Muscles
10. Glandular structures – lymph and salivary

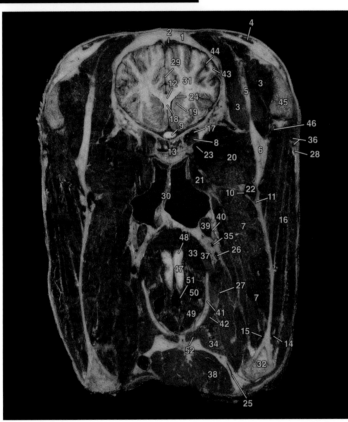

1 **Parietal bone**
2 **Dorsal sagittal sinus**
3 Temporalis m.
4 Frontoscutularis m.
5 **Coronoid process of mandible**
6 **Mandibular ramus**
7 Medial pterygoid m.
8 Maxillary branch of trigeminal n. (alar canal)
9 Optic chiasm
10 **Inferior alveolar a.**
11 Inferior alveolar n.
12 Corpus callosum
13 **Presphenoid bone and sphenopalatine sinus**
14 **Ventral masseteric v. and masseteric branches of external carotid a.**
15 **Pterygoid branches of facial a. and v.**
16 Masseter m.

17 Oculomotor n., trochlear n., abducens n., and ophthalmic n. (in orbital fissure)
18 Septum pellucidum
19 Caudate nucleus
20 Lateral pterygoid m.
21 Tensor muscle of soft palate
22 **Maxillary v.**
23 **Maxillary a.**
24 Lateral ventricle
25 **Linguofacial v.**
26 **Linguofacial trunk**
27 Digastricus tendon (caudal belly)
28 Facial n., buccal branch
29 Falx cerebri
30 Septum of auditory diverticula (guttural pouches)
31 Cerebral cortex (white matter tracts)
32 **Mandible**
33 Palatopharyngeus m.
34 **Mandibular salivary gland**

35 Ascending palatine a.
36 Transverse facial a. and v.
37 Hyopharyngeus m.
38 Omohyoideus and sternohyoideus mm.
39 Stylopharyngeus m.
40 **Stylohyoid bone**
41 Thyroid cartilage
42 Thyrohyoideus m.
43 Cerebral gyrus
44 Cerebral sulcus
45 **Zygomatic process of temporal bone**
46 **Superficial temporalis v., a., and masseteric n.**
47 Arytenoid cartilage
48 Corniculate process of arytenoid cartilage
49 Ventricularis m.
50 Laryngeal ventricle
51 Vocal cord
52 Cricothyroideus m.

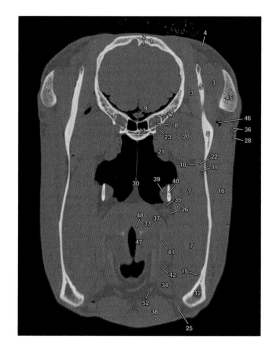

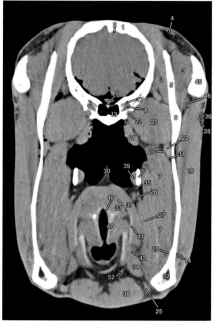

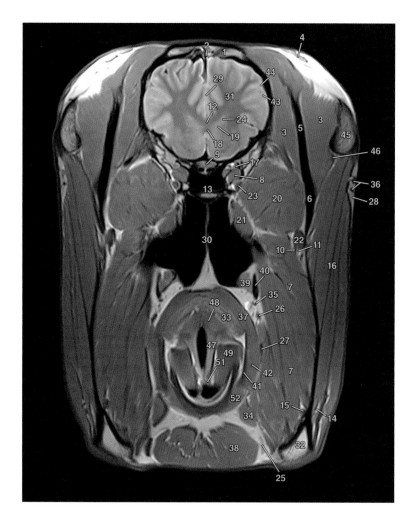

T29

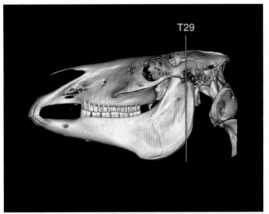

1. Bones of the head
2. Oral and dental structures
3. Nasal and sinus structures
4. Larynx, pharynx, and guttural pouches
5. Ophthalmic structures
6. Auricular structures
7. Brain and nervous system
8. Vascular anatomy
9. Muscles
10. Glandular structures – lymph and salivary

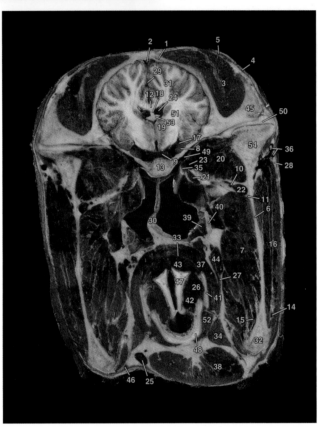

1 Parietal bone	18 Septum pellucidum	**36 Transverse facial a. and v.**
2 Dorsal sagittal sinus	19 Caudate nucleus	37 Thyropharyngeus m.
3 Temporalis m.	20 Lateral pterygoid m.	38 Omohyoideus and sternohyoideus mm.
4 Frontoscutularis m.	21 Tensor muscle of soft palate	39 Stylopharyngeus m.
5 Interscutularis m.	**22 Maxillary v.**	**40 Stylohyoid bone**
6 Mandibular ramus	**23 Maxillary a.**	41 Thyroid cartilage
7 Medial pterygoid m.	24 Lateral ventricle with choroid plexus	42 Vocalis m.
8 Maxillary branch of trigeminal n.	**25 Linguofacial v.**	43 Transverse arytenoideus m.
9 Optic chiasm	26 Lateral cricoarytenoideus m.	44 Stylohyoideus m.
10 Inferior alveolar a.	27 Digastricus tendon	**45 Zygomatic process of temporal bone**
11 Inferior alveolar n.	28 Facial n., buccal branch	**46 Parotid duct**
12 Corpus callosum	29 Falx cerebri	47 Arytenoid cartilage
13 Basisphenoid bone	30 Septum of diverticulum of the auditory	48 Cricoid cartilage
14 Ventral masseteric v. and masseteric	tube (guttural pouch)	**49 Subtemporal venous plexus**
branches of external carotid a.	31 Corona radiata	50 Articular disk
15 Pterygoid branches of facial a. and v.	**32 Mandible**	51 Internal capsule
16 Masseter m.	33 Palatopharyngeus m.	52 Cricothyroideus m.
17 Oculomotor n., trochlear n., abducens n.,	**34 Mandibular salivary gland**	53 Fornix
and ophthalmic n.	35 Levator muscle of soft palate	**54 Condylar process of the mandible**

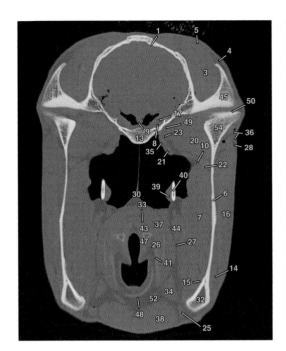

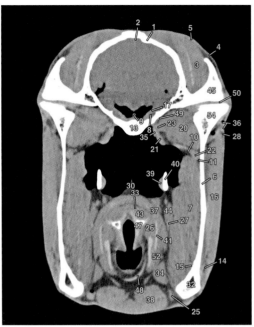

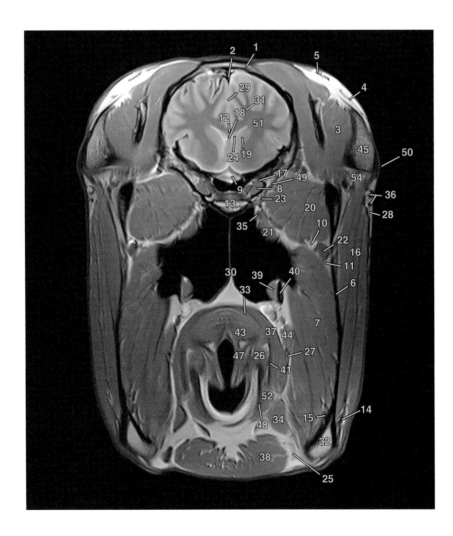

T30

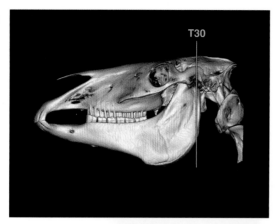

1. Bones of the head
2. Oral and dental structures
3. Nasal and sinus structures
4. Larynx, pharynx, and guttural pouches
5. Ophthalmic structures
6. Auricular structures
7. Brain and nervous system
8. Vascular anatomy
9. Muscles
10. Glandular structures – lymph and salivary

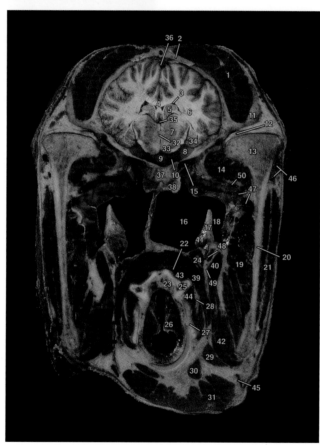

1 Temporalis m.	18 Auditory diverticulum (guttural pouch) lateral compartment	35 Third ventricle
2 Parietal bone	19 Medial pterygoid m.	**36 Dorsal sagittal sinus**
3 Lateral ventricle	**20 Ramus of the mandible**	**37 Basisphenoid bone**
4 Corpus callosum	21 Massester m.	38 Longus capitis m.
5 Hippocampus	22 Cricoarytenoideus dorsalis m.	39 Thyropharyngeus m.
6 Internal capsule	23 Arytenoid cartilage	40 Stylohyoideus m.
7 Thalamus	**24 Medial retropharyngeal lymph node**	41 Stylopharyngeus m.
8 Trigeminal n.	25 Arytenoid cartilage, articular surface	42 Digastricus m. (occipitomandibular part)
9 Hypophysis	26 Arytenoid cartilage, vocal process	43 Transverse arytenoideus m.
10 Cavernous venous sinus	27 Cricoid cartilage	44 Lateral cricoarytenoideus m.
11 Zygomatic process of temporal bone	28 Thyroid cartilage, caudal cornu	**45 Linguofacial v.**
12 Articular disk	29 Mandibular salivary gland	**46 Transverse facial a. and v.**
13 Condylar process of the mandible	30 Sternothyroideus m.	**47 Maxillary v. and inferior alveolar a.**
14 Lateral pterygoid m.	31 Sternohyoideus and omohyoideus mm.	**48 Linguofacial trunk**
15 Subtemporal venous plexus	32 Interthalamic adhesion	**49 Lateral retropharyngeal lymph node**
16 Auditory diverticulum (guttural pouch), medial compartment	33 Hypothalamus	**50 Maxillary a.**
17 Stylohyoid bone	34 Piriform lobe	

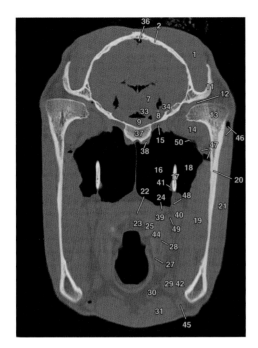

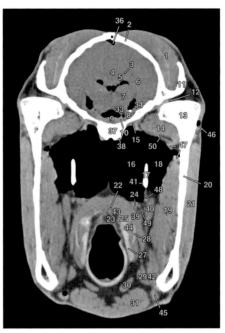

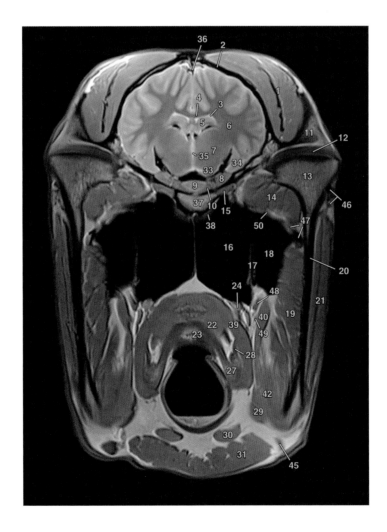

T31

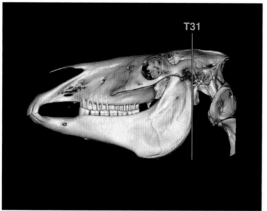

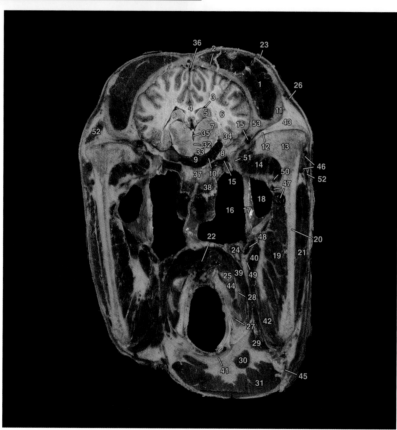

1 Temporalis m.	18 Auditory tube diverticulum (guttural pouch), lateral compartment	36 Dorsal sagittal sinus
2 Parietal bone	**19 Medial pterygoid m.**	**37 Basisphenoid bone**
3 Lateral ventricle	**20 Ramus of the mandible**	38 Longus capitis m.
4 Corpus callosum	21 Masseter m.	39 Cricopharyngeus m.
5 Hippocampus	22 Cricoarytenoideus dorsalis m.	40 Stylohyoideus m.
6 Internal capsule	23 Frontoscutularis m.	41 First tracheal cartilage
7 Thalamus	**24 Medial retropharyngeal lymph node**	42 Digastricus m. (occipitomandibular part)
8 Trigeminal n.	25 Arytenoid cartilage, articular surface	**43 Caudal compartment of the dorsal synovial pouch (intraarticular fat)**
9 Hypophysis	26 Zygomaticoscutularis m.	44 Lateral cricoarytenoideus m.
10 Cavernous venous sinus	27 Cricoid cartilage	**45 Linguofacial v.**
11 Zygomatic process of temporal bone	28 Thyroid cartilage, caudal cornu	**46 Transverse facial a. and v.**
12 Articular disk	**29 Mandibular salivary gland**	**47 Maxillary v. and inferior alveolar a.**
13 Condylar process of the mandible	30 Sternothyroideus m.	**48 Linguofacial trunk and maxillary a.**
14 Lateral pterygoid m.	31 Sternohyoideus and omohyoideus mm.	**49 Lateral retropharyngeal lymph node**
15 Ventral petrous venous sinus	32 Interthalamic adhesion	**50 Maxillary a.**
16 Auditory tube diverticulum (guttural pouch), medial compartment	33 Hypothalamus	51 Mandibular n.
	34 Piriform lobe	**52 Parotid salivary gland**
17 Stylohyoid bone	35 Third ventricle	**53 Squamous portion of the temporal bone**

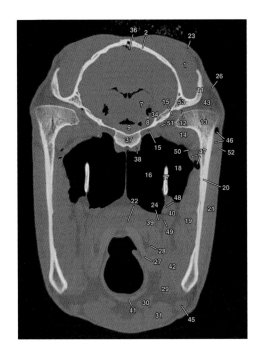
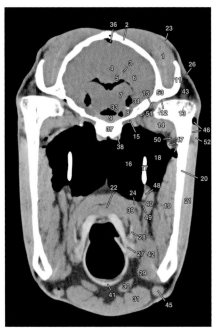
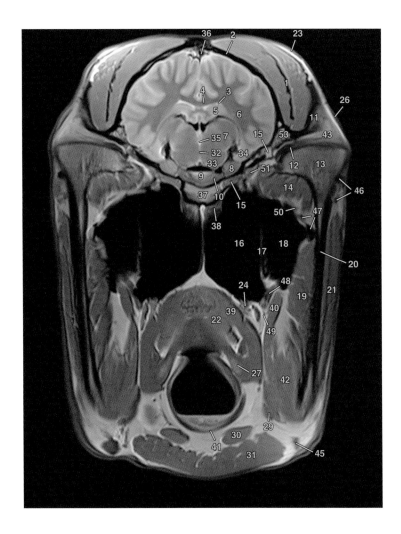

T32

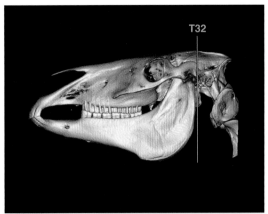

1. **Bones of the head**
2. Oral and dental structures
3. **Nasal and sinus structures**
4. Larynx, pharynx, and guttural pouches
5. Ophthalmic structures
6. **Auricular structures**
7. Brain and nervous system
8. **Vascular anatomy**
9. Muscles
10. **Glandular structures – lymph and salivary**

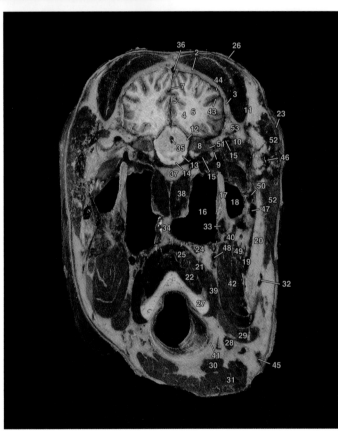

1 Temporalis m.
2 Parietal bone
3 Squamous suture
4 Corpus callosum
5 Cingulate gyrus
6 Internal capsule
7 Falx cerebri
8 Trigeminal n.
9 Foramen lacerum
10 Articular tubercle of the temporal bone
11 Zygomatic process of the temporal bone
12 Rostral colliculus
13 Crus cerebri
14 Transverse pontine fibers
15 Ventral petrous venous sinus
16 Auditory diverticulum (guttural pouch), medial compartment
17 Stylohyoid bone

18 Auditory diverticulum (guttural pouch), lateral compartment
19 Medial pterygoid m.
20 Ramus of the mandible
21 Thyropharyngeus m.
22 Cricoarytenoideus dorsalis m.
23 Parotidoauricularis m.
24 Medial retropharyngeal lymph node
25 Esophagus
26 Interscutularis m.
27 Cricoid cartilage
28 Thyroid gland
29 Mandibular salivary gland
30 Sternothyroideus m.
31 Sternohyoideus and omohyoideus mm.
32 Ventral masseteric v. and a.
33 Occipitohyoideus m.
34 Septum of diverticula of the auditory tube (guttural pouch)

35 Mesencephalic aqueduct
36 Dorsal sagittal sinus
37 Basisphenoid bone
38 Longus capitis m.
39 Cricopharyngeus m.
40 Stylohyoideus m.
41 Tracheal cartilage
42 Digastricus m. (occipitomandibular part)
43 Sulcus
44 Gyrus
45 Linguofacial v.
46 Superficial temporalis v.
47 Maxillary v.
48 External carotid a.
49 Lateral retropharyngeal lymph node
50 Maxillary a.
51 Mandibular n. (branching from trigeminal n.)
52 Parotid salivary gland
53 Squamous portion of the temporal bone

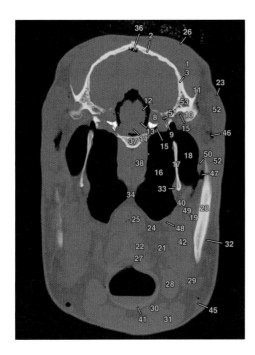

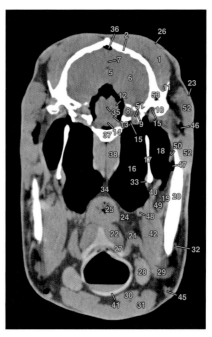

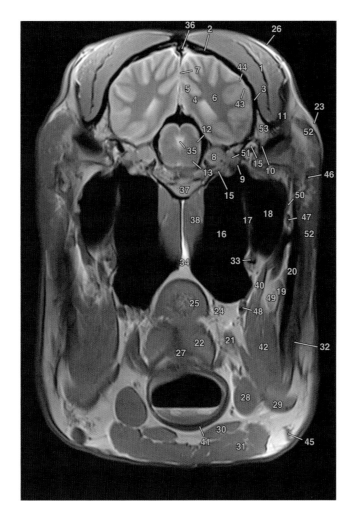

T33

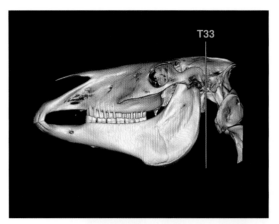

1. **Bones of the head**
2. **Oral and dental structures**
3. **Nasal and sinus structures**
4. Larynx, pharynx, and guttural pouches
5. **Ophthalmic structures**
6. **Auricular structures**
7. Brain and nervous system
8. **Vascular anatomy**
9. Muscles
10. **Glandular structures – lymph and salivary**

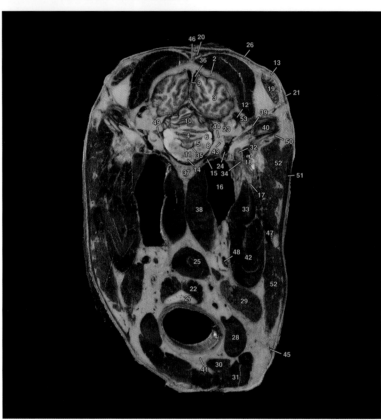

1 Temporalis m.	18 Diverticulum of the auditory tube (guttural pouch), lateral compartment	35 Fourth ventricle
2 Parietal bone	19 Deep scutuloauricularis m.	**36 Dorsal sagittal sinus**
3 Occipital lobe of cerebrum	20 Parietoauricular m.	**37 Basilar part of occipital bone**
4 Pars rostralis (cerebellum)	21 Ventral superficial scutuloauricularis m.	38 Longus capitis m.
5 Rostral cerebellar peduncle	22 Cricoarytenoideus dorsalis m.	39 External acoustic opening
6 Middle cerebellar peduncle	**23 Petrous part of temporal bone**	40 External auditory meatus
7 Tentorium cerebelli osseum	**24 Tympanic cavity of the temporal bone (middle ear)**	41 Tracheal cartilage
8 Trigeminal nerve root	25 Esophagus	42 Digastricus m. (occipitomandibular part)
9 Falx cerebri	26 Dorsal superficial scutuloauricularis m.	43 Cochlea of the inner ear
10 Pars caudalis (cerebellum)	27 Cricoid cartilage	**44 Internal acoustic meatus**
11 Medulla oblongata	**28 Thyroid gland**	**45 Linguofacial v.**
12 Dorsal cerebral v.	**29 Mandibular salivary gland**	**46 External sagittal crest**
13 Scutiform cartilage	30 Sternothyroideus m.	**47 Maxillary v.**
14 Pyramidal tract	31 Sternohyoideus and omohyoideus mm.	**48 External carotid a.**
15 Foramen lacerum emissary v.	**32 Styloid process of the temporal bone**	49 Facial and vestibulocochlear nn.
16 Diverticulum of the auditory tube (guttural pouch), medial compartment	33 Occipitohyoideus m.	**50 Auricular cartilage**
17 Stylohyoid bone (caudal aspect)	**34 Tympanohyoideum**	51 Parotidoauricularis m.
		52 Parotid salivary gland
		53 Squamous portion of the temporal bone

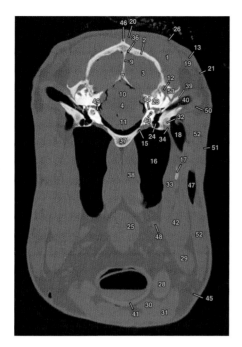

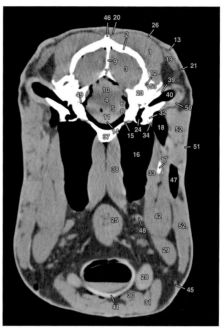

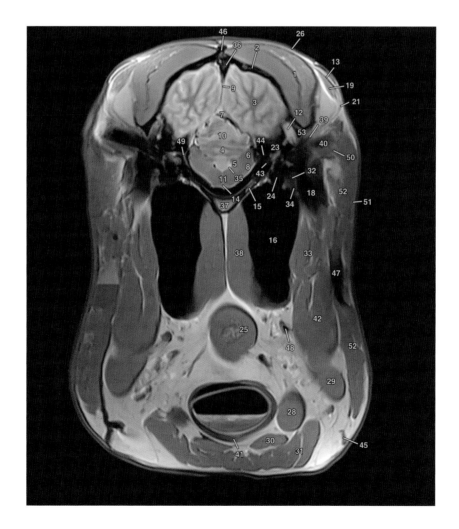

T34

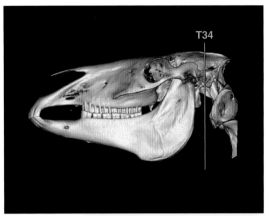

1. **Bones of the head**
2. Oral and dental structures
3. **Nasal and sinus structures**
4. Larynx, pharynx, and guttural pouches
5. Ophthalmic structures
6. **Auricular structures**
7. Brain and nervous system
8. **Vascular anatomy**
9. Muscles
10. **Glandular structures – lymph and salivary**

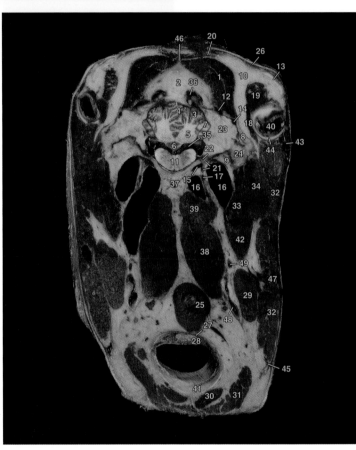

1 Temporalis m.	18 Minor deep cervicoauricularis m.	34 Obliquus capitis cranialis m.
2 Occipital bone	19 Deep scutuloauricularis m.	35 Choroid plexus in fourth ventricle
3 Cerebellar hemisphere	20 Parietoauricularis m.	**36 Transverse venous sinus**
4 Vermis cerebelli	21 Vagus, internal carotid, glossopharyngeal,	**37 Basilar part of occipital bone**
5 Cerebellar white matter	and accessory nn.	38 Longus capitis m.
6 Nodulus	**22 Jugular foramen**	39 Rectus capitis ventralis m.
7 Paraflocculus	**23 Petrous part of temporal bone**	**40 External auditory meatus**
8 Squamous part of temporal bone	**24 Mastoid process of temporal bone**	41 Tracheal cartilage
9 Paracondylar (jugular) process	25 Esophagus	42 Digastricus m. (occipitomandibular part)
10 Auricular adipose body	26 Dorsal superficial scutuloauricularis m.	43 Parotidoauricularis m.
11 Medulla oblongata	27 Membranous wall (dorsal ends of	**44 Auricular cartilage**
12 Dorsal cerebral v.	tracheal cartilage do not meet)	**45 Linguofacial v.**
13 Scutiform cartilage	28 Trachealis m.	**46 External sagittal crest**
14 Caudal meningeal a.	**29 Mandibular salivary gland**	**47 Maxillary v.**
15 Foramen lacerum emissary v.	30 Sternothyroideus m.	**48 Common carotid a.**
16 Auditory diverticulum (guttural pouch),	31 Sternohyoideus and omohyoideus mm.	**49 Occipital a.**
medial compartment	**32 Parotid salivary gland**	
17 Internal carotid a.	33 Occipitohyoideus m.	

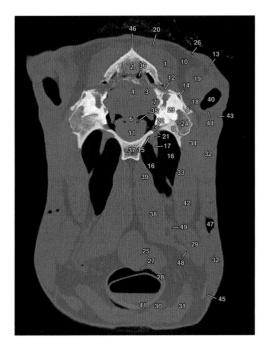

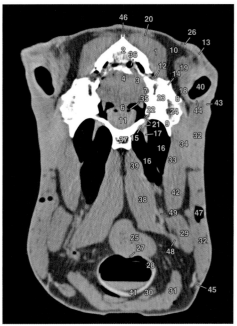

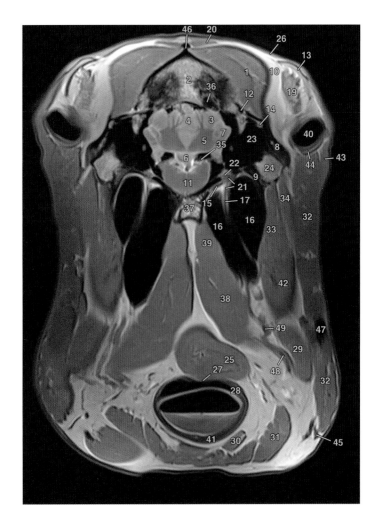

T35

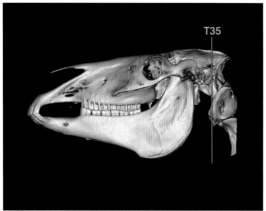

1. **Bones of the head**
2. Oral and dental structures
3. **Nasal and sinus structures**
4. Larynx, pharynx, and guttural pouches
5. **Ophthalmic structures**
6. **Auricular structures**
7. Brain and nervous system
8. **Vascular anatomy**
9. Muscles
10. **Glandular structures – lymph and salivary**

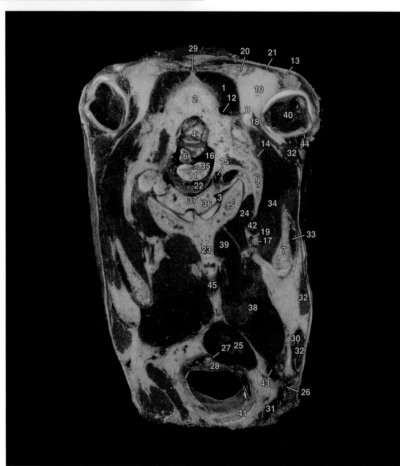

1 Temporalis m.	16 Foramen magnum	31 Sternohyoideus and omohyoideus mm.
2 Occipital bone	17 Occipital a.	32 Parotid salivary gland
3 Atlantooccipital joint	18 Minor deep cervicoauricularis m.	33 Obliquus capitis caudalis m.
4 Vermis cerebelli	19 Occipital artery branch	34 Obliquus capitis cranialis m.
5 Atlas	20 Parietoauricularis m.	35 Central canal of the spinal cord
6 Nodulus	21 Superficial cervicoauricularis m.	36 Occipital condyle
7 Transverse process (atlas)	22 Subarachnoid space	37 Basilar part of occipital bone
8 Supramastoid crest	23 Ventral tubercle (atlas)	38 Longus capitis m.
9 Paracondylar (jugular) process	24 Rectus capitis lateralis m.	39 Rectus capitis ventralis m.
10 Auricular adipose body	25 Esophagus	40 External auditory meatus
11 Cranial cervical spinal cord	26 External jugular v.	41 Tracheal cartilage
12 Dorsal cerebral v.	27 Membranous wall of the trachea (dorsal	42 Digastricus m. (occipitomandibular part)
13 Scutiform cartilage	ends of tracheal cartilage do not meet)	43 Common carotid a.
14 Caudal meningeal a.	28 Trachealis m.	44 Auricular cartilage
15 Occipital emissary v. (in condyloid	29 External sagittal crest	45 Longus colli m.
canal)	30 Maxillary v.	

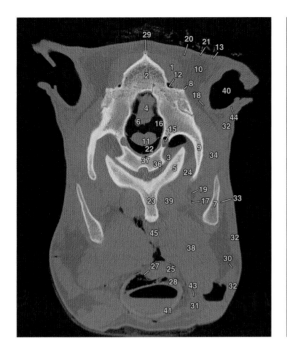

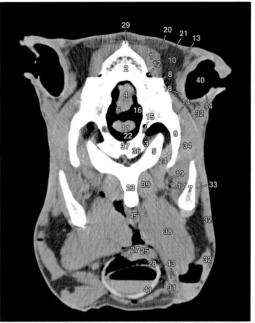

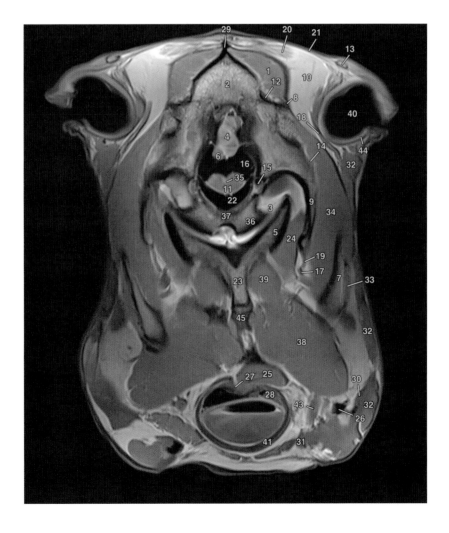

T36

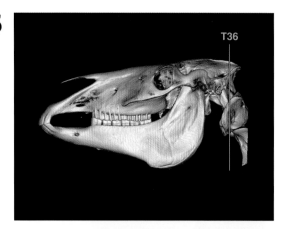

1. **Bones of the head**
2. Oral and dental structures
3. **Nasal and sinus structures**
4. Larynx, pharynx, and guttural pouches
5. **Ophthalmic structures**
6. **Auricular structures**
7. Brain and nervous system
8. **Vascular anatomy**
9. Muscles
10. **Glandular structures – lymph and salivary**

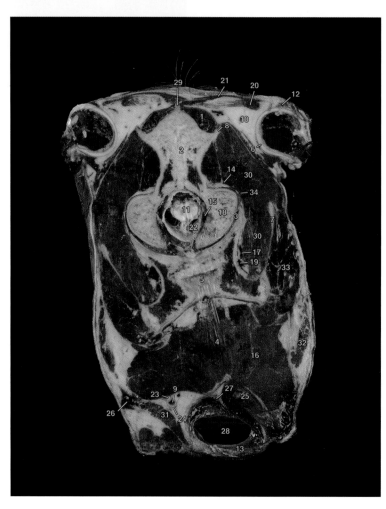

1 Temporalis m.
2 **Occipital bone**
3 **Atlantooccipital joint**
4 Longus colli m.
5 **Atlas**
6 Auricular cartilage
7 **Transverse process (atlas)**
8 **Temporal crest**
9 **Common carotid a.**
10 **Auricular adipose body**
11 Cervical spinal cord
12 Superficial scutuloauricularis m.

13 Tracheal cartilage
14 **Caudal meningeal a.**
15 Occipital emissary v.
16 Longus capitis m.
17 **Occipital a.**
18 **Occipital condyle**
19 **Occipital v.**
20 Parietoauricularis m.
21 Superficial cervicoauricularis m.
22 Subarachnoid space
23 Vagosympathetic trunk
24 Recurrent laryngeal n.

25 Esophagus
26 **External jugular v.**
27 Membranous wall (dorsal ends of tracheal cartilage do not meet)
28 Tracheal lumen
29 **External sagittal crest**
30 Obliquus capitis cranialis m.
31 Sternohyoideus and omohyoideus mm.
32 Brachiocephalicus m.
33 Obliquus capitis caudalis m.
34 **Atlantooccipital joint capsule**

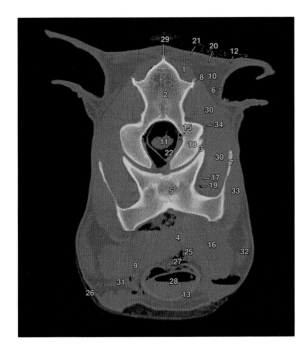

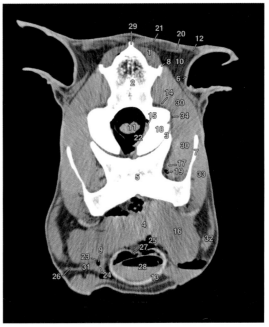

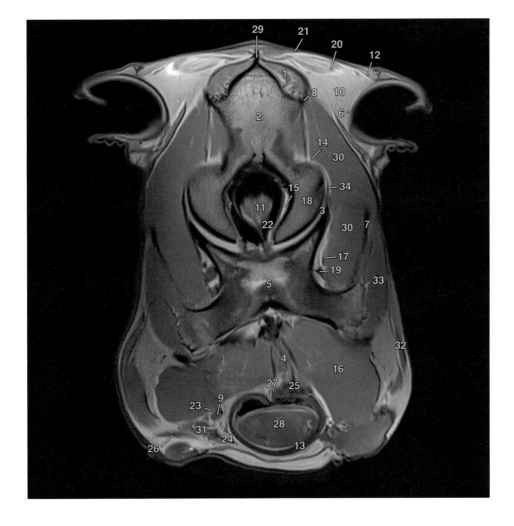

T37

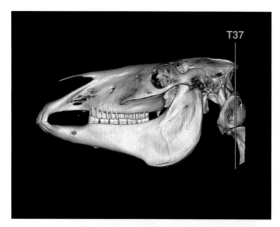

1. **Bones of the head**
2. Oral and dental structures
3. **Nasal and sinus structures**
4. Larynx, pharynx, and guttural pouches
5. **Ophthalmic structures**
6. **Auricular structures**
7. Brain and nervous system
8. **Vascular anatomy**
9. Muscles
10. **Glandular structures – lymph and salivary**

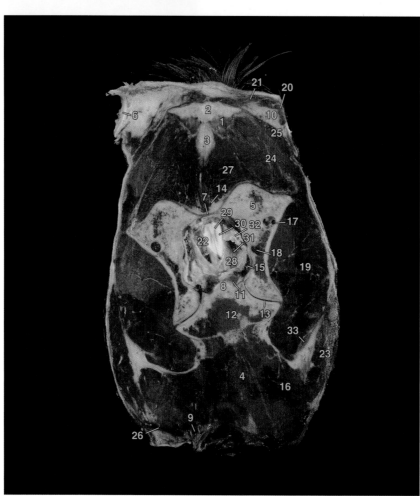

1 Semispinalis m. insertion	**12 Axis (C2)**	23 Brachiocephalicus m.
2 Nuchal crest (occipital bone)	**13 Atlanto-occipital joint**	24 Obliquus capitis cranialis m.
3 Nuchal ligament (funicular portion)	**14 Caudal meningeal a.**	25 Splenius m.
4 Longus colli m.	**15 Internal vertebral plexus**	**26 External jugular v.**
5 Atlas (C1)	16 Longus capitis m.	27 Rectus capitis dorsalis m.
6 Auricular cartilage	**17 Vertebral a., v. and n. in alar foramen**	28 Spinal dura mater
7 Dorsal atlanto-occipital membrane	**18 Nutrient foramen**	29 Gray matter of the spinal cord
8 Dens of axis	19 Obliquus capitis caudalis m.	30 White matter of the spinal cord
9 Common carotid a.	20 Deep cervicoauricularis m.	31 Epidural space
10 Auricular adipose body	21 Superficial cervicoauricularis m.	32 Epidural fat
11 Alar ligaments	22 Subarachnoid space	33 Longissimus atlantis m.

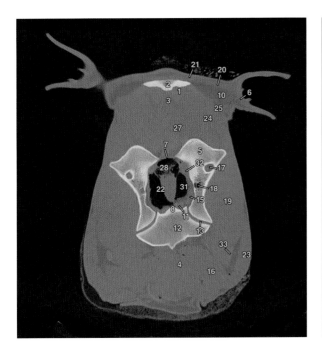

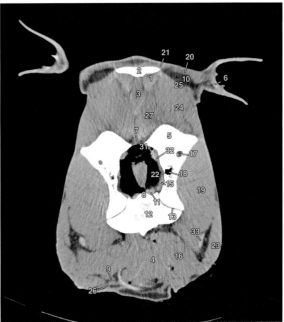

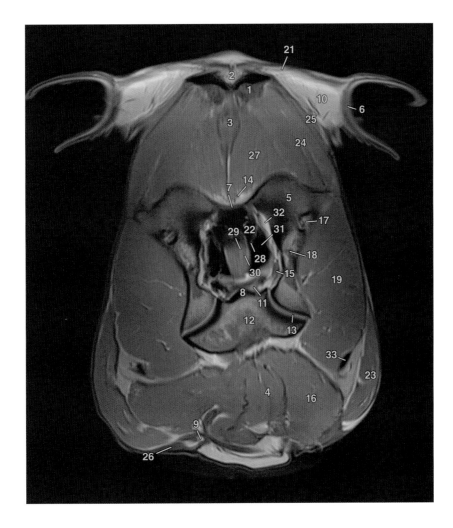

CHAPTER 3

Clinical and Surgical Anatomy of the Equine Head: Sagittal Sections

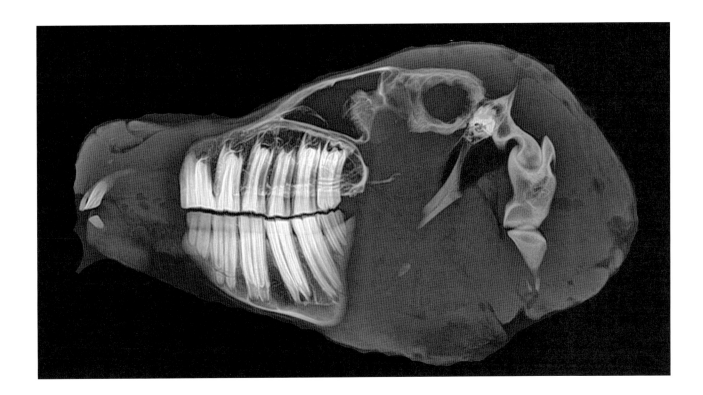

Atlas of Clinical Imaging and Anatomy of the Equine Head, First Edition. Larry Kimberlin, Alex zur Linden and Lynn Ruoff.
© 2017 John Wiley & Sons, Inc. Published 2017 by John Wiley & Sons, Inc.

S1

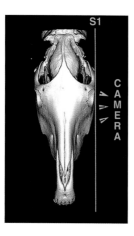

1. **Bones of the head**
2. **Oral and dental structures**
3. **Nasal and sinus structures**
4. Larynx, pharynx, and guttural pouches
5. **Ophthalmic structures**
6. **Auricular structures**
7. Brain and nervous system
8. **Vascular anatomy**
9. Muscles
10. **Glandular structures – lymph and salivary**

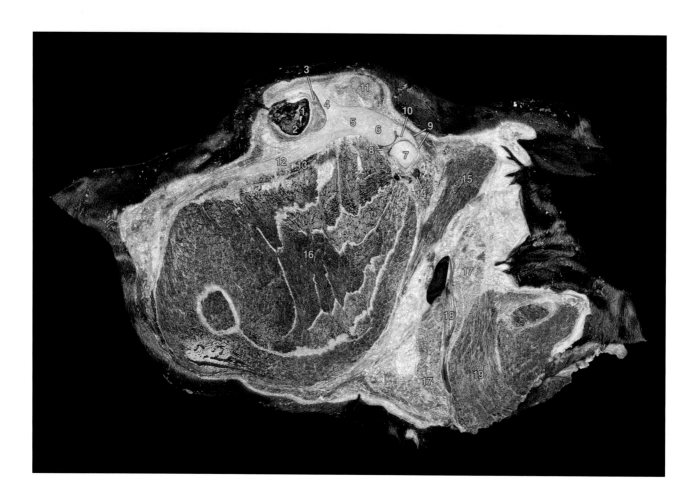

1 Vitreous body	9 Articular capsule	15 Digastricus m.
2 Lens	10 Caudal compartment of the dorsal synovial pouch of the temporomandibular joint	16 Masseter m.
3 Lacrimal gland		17 **Parotid salivary gland**
4 Zygomatic process of the frontal bone		18 **Maxillary vein**
5 Zygomatic bone	11 Adipose body of temporal fossa	19 Brachiocephalicus m.
6 Zygomatic process of the temporal bone	12 Facial crest of the maxillary and zygomatic bones	
7 Condylar process of the mandible	13 Transverse facial sinus	
8 Articular disk of the temporomandibular joint	14 Transverse facial vein	

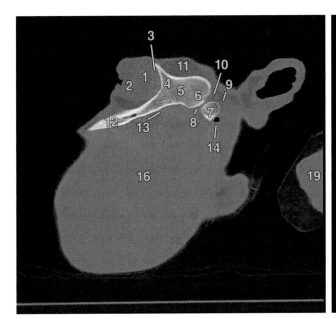

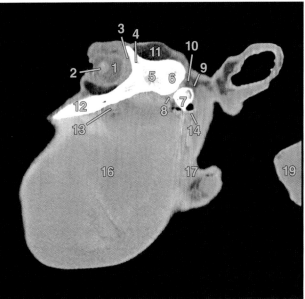

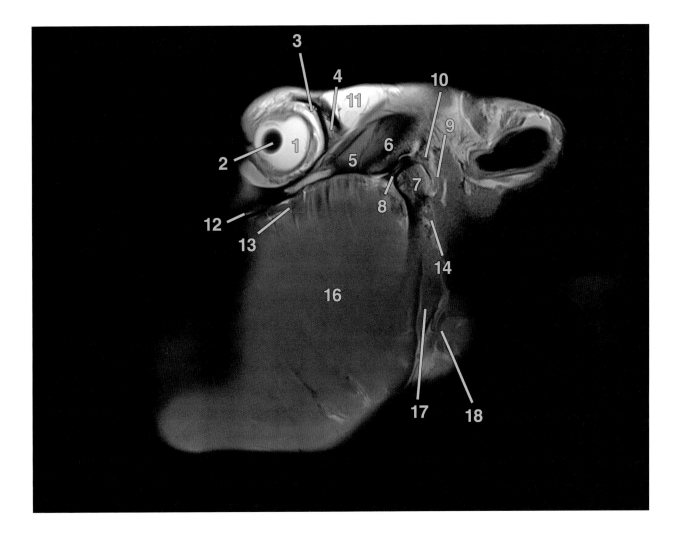

S2

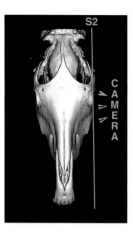

1. **Bones of the head**
2. Oral and dental structures
3. **Nasal and sinus structures**
4. Larynx, pharynx, and guttural pouches
5. Ophthalmic structures
6. Auricular structures
7. Brain and nervous system
8. **Vascular anatomy**
9. Muscles
10. **Glandular structures – lymph and salivary**

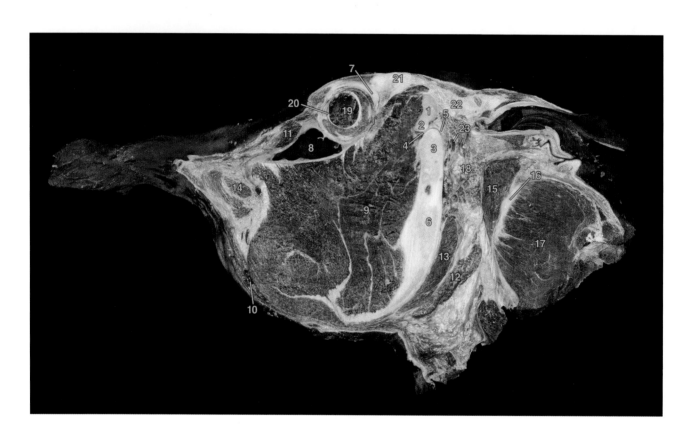

1 Zygomatic process of the temporal bone	8 Maxillary sinus – caudal portion	17 Obliquus capitis caudalis m.
2 Articular tubercle	9 Masseter m.	18 Parotid salivary gland
3 Condylar process of the mandible	10 Facial v.	19 Vitreal chamber
4 Articular disk of the temporomandibular joint	11 Levator labii superioris m.	20 Sclera
5 Caudal fibrous expansion of the articular disk	12 Mandibular salivary gland	21 Adipose body of temporal fossa
6 Ramus of the mandible	13 Digastricus m.	22 Auricular adipose body
7 Frontal bone	14 Buccinator m.	23 Superficial temporal v.
	15 Obliquus capitis cranialis m.	
	16 Wing of the atlas (C1)	

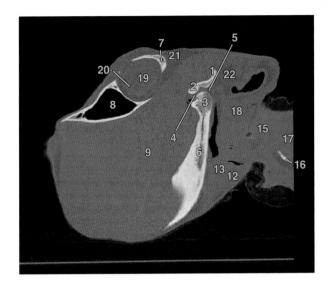

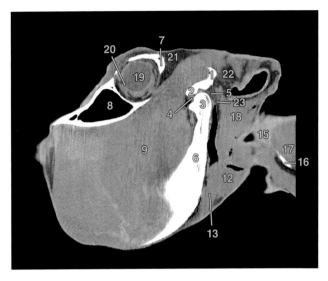

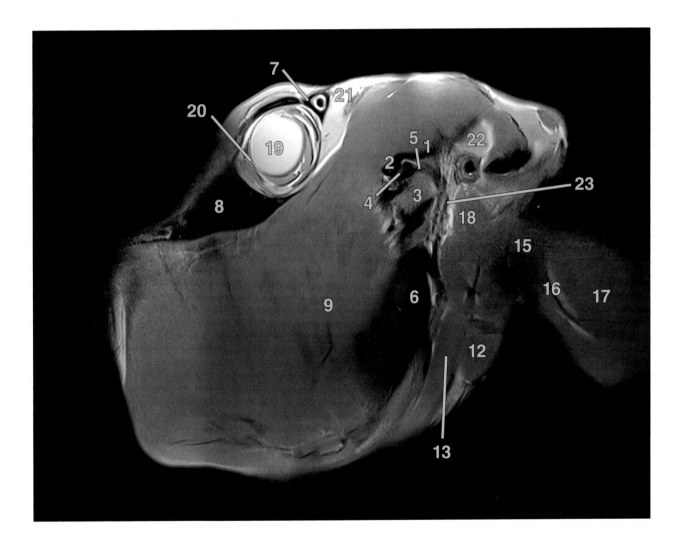

S3

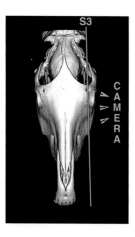

1. Bones of the head
2. Oral and dental structures
3. Nasal and sinus structures
4. Larynx, pharynx, and guttural pouches
5. Ophthalmic structures
6. Auricular structures
7. Brain and nervous system
8. Vascular anatomy
9. Muscles
10. Glandular structures – lymph and salivary

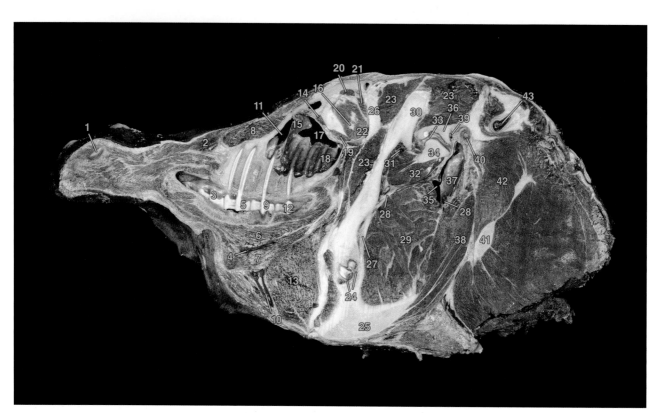

1 Alar cartilage	15 Maxillary sinus septum	30 Coronoid process of the mandible
2 Levator nasolabialis m.	16 Optic n.	31 Masseteric v.
3 Crown of tooth 207 (left superior third premolar)	17 Caudal maxillary sinus	32 Lateral pterygoid m.
4 Inferior labialis v.	18 Alveolar bone and sinus epithelium covering root of tooth 211 (left superior third molar)	33 Articular disk of the temporomandibular joint
5 Crown of tooth 208 (left superior fourth premolar)	19 Ventral rectus m.	34 Condylar process of the mandible
6 Buccinator m.	20 Dorsal oblique m.	35 Diverticulum of the auditory tube (guttural pouch), lateral compartment
7 Depressor labii inferioris m.	21 Dorsal rectus m.	36 Mandibular fossa of the temporal bone
8 Levator labii superioris m.	22 Retractor bulbi m.	37 Diverticulum of the auditory tube (guttural pouch) epithelium covering the stylohyoid bone
9 Crown of tooth 209 (left superior first molar)	23 Temporalis m.	
10 Facial v.	24 Root of tooth 311 (left inferior third molar)	38 Digastricus m.
11 Rostral maxillary sinus	25 Angle of the mandible	39 Temporal venous sinus
12 Crown of tooth 210 (left superior second molar)	26 Orbital portion of the frontal bone	40 External auditory meatus
13 Masseter m.	27 Inferior alveolar v. (in mandibular canal)	41 Wing of the atlas
14 Ventral oblique m.	28 Maxillary v.	42 Obliquus capitis cranialis m.
	29 Medial pterygoid m.	43 External ear canal

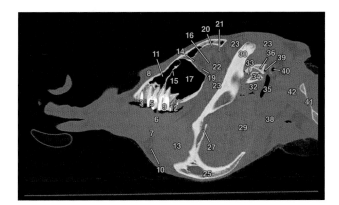

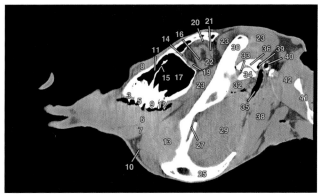

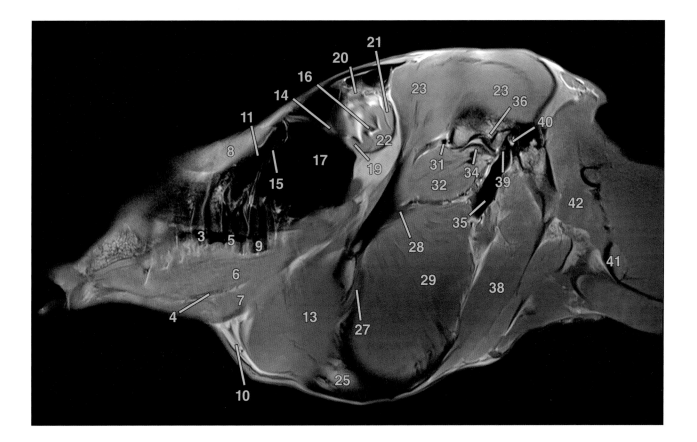

S4

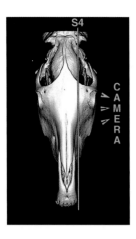

1. **Bones of the head**
2. **Oral and dental structures**
3. **Nasal and sinus structures**
4. Larynx, pharynx, and guttural pouches
5. **Ophthalmic structures**
6. **Auricular structures**
7. Brain and nervous system
8. **Vascular anatomy**
9. Muscles
10. **Glandular structures – lymph and salivary**

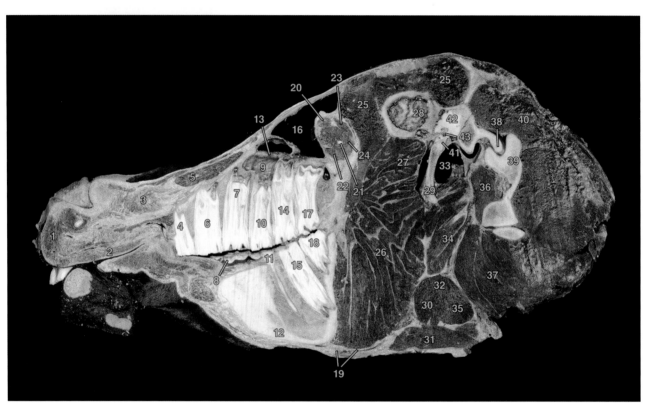

1 Superior incisor m.	13 Infraorbital canal	27 Lateral pterygoid m.
2 Orbicularis oris m.	14 Root of tooth 210 (left superior second molar)	28 Temporal lobe of the cerebrum
3 Levator nasolabialis m.		29 **Stylohyoid bone**
4 Root of tooth 206 (left superior second premolar)	15 Root of tooth 310 (left inferior second molar)	30 Hyopharyngeus m.
5 Levator labii superioris m. (aka levator labii maxillaris)	16 **Conchofrontal sinus**	31 Sternohyoideus and omohyoideus mm.
	17 Root of tooth 211 (left superior third molar)	32 Thyropharyngeal m.
6 Root of tooth 207 (left superior third premolar)	18 Root of tooth 311 (left inferior third molar)	33 Auditory diverticulum (guttural pouch), medial compartment
7 Root of tooth 208 (left superior fourth premolar)	19 **Facial v.**	34 Digastricus m.
8 Crown of tooth 308 (left inferior fourth premolar)	20 Dorsal oblique m.	35 Cricopharyngeal m.
	21 Optic n.	36 Rectus capitis ventralis m.
9 **Rostral maxillary sinus**	22 Ventral rectus m.	37 Longus capitis m.
10 Root of tooth 209 (left superior first molar)	23 Dorsal rectus m.	38 **Occipital condyle**
11 Crown of tooth 309 (left inferior first molar)	24 Retractor bulbi m.	39 **Atlas**
	25 Temporalis m.	40 Obliquus capitis cranialis m.
12 **Border of the mandible**	26 Medial pterygoid m.	41 **Tympanohyoideum**
		42 **Temporal bone (petrous portion)**
		43 **Tympanic cavity**

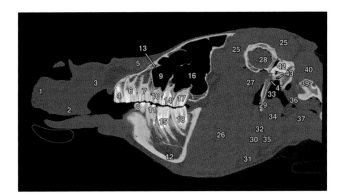

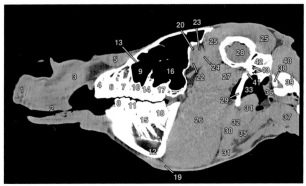

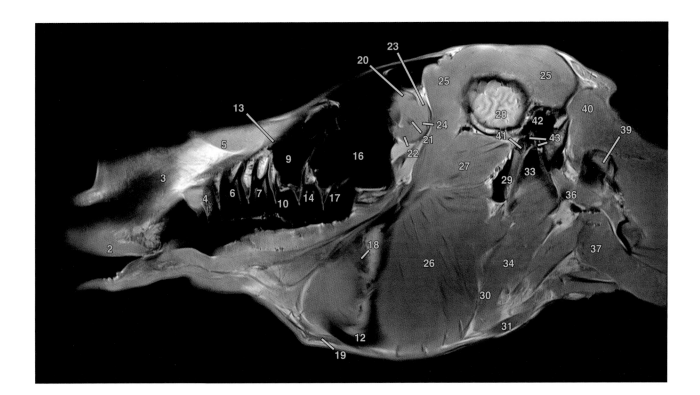

S5

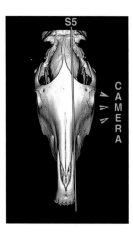

1. **Bones of the head**
2. **Oral and dental structures**
3. **Nasal and sinus structures**
4. Larynx, pharynx, and guttural pouches
5. **Ophthalmic structures**
6. **Auricular structures**
7. Brain and nervous system
8. **Vascular anatomy**
9. Muscles
10. **Glandular structures – lymph and salivary**

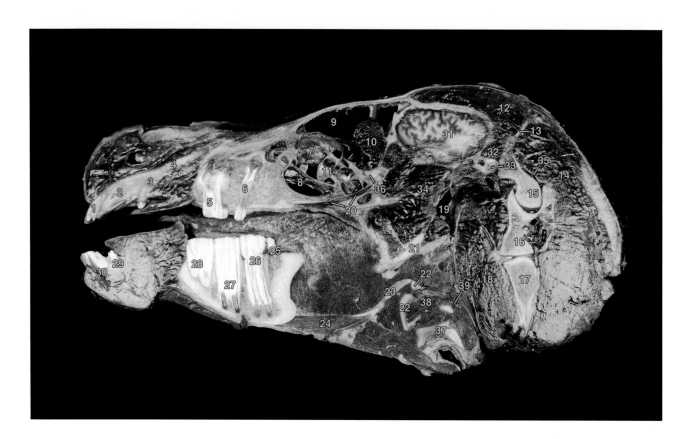

1 Tooth 202 (left superior intermediate incisor)	13 Lateral portion of the occipital bone	28 Tooth 306 (left inferior second premolar)
2 Tooth 203 (left superior corner incisor)	14 Obliquus capitis cranialis m.	29 Tooth 304 (left inferior canine tooth)
3 Tooth 204 (left superior canine tooth)	15 Condyle of the occipital bone	30 Tooth 303 (left inferior corner incisor)
4 Incisive bone	16 Atlas	31 Temporal lobe (cerebrum)
5 Root of tooth 206 (left superior second premolar)	17 Axis	32 Cerebellum (lateral aspect)
6 Root of tooth 207 (left superior third premolar)	18 Longus capitis m.	33 Vestibule (in petrous part of temporal bone)
7 Dorsal nasal concha	19 Guttural pouch	34 Lateral pterygoid m.
8 Ventral nasal meatus	20 Greater palantine v.	35 Joint capsule (atlantooccipital joint)
9 Conchofrontal sinus	21 Stylohyoid bone	36 Infraorbital n.
10 Ethmoidal labyrinth	22 Thyroid cartilage	37 Cricoid cartilage
11 Roots of teeth 210 and 211 (left superior second and third molars)	23 Thyrohyoid bone	38 Lateral cricoarytenoideus m.
12 Temporalis m.	24 Geniohyoideus m.	39 Cricoarytenoideus dorsalis m.
	25 Tooth 309 (left inferior first molar)	
	26 Tooth 308 (left inferior fourth premolar)	
	27 Tooth 407 (left inferior third premolar)	

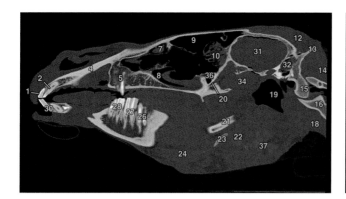

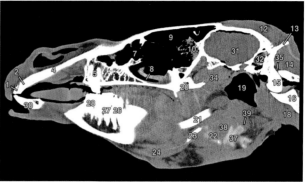

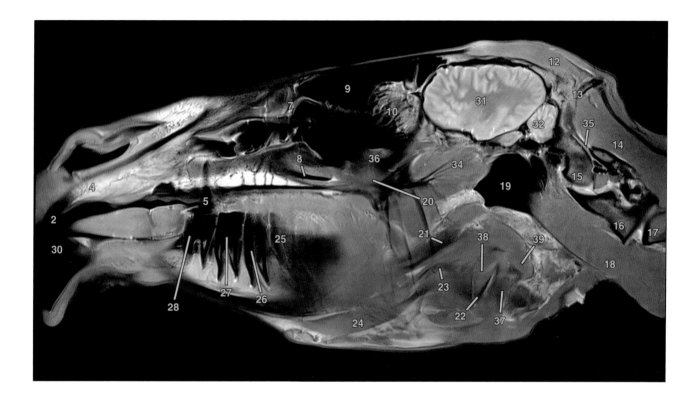

S6

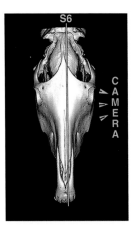

1. **Bones of the head**
2. **Oral and dental structures**
3. **Nasal and sinus structures**
4. Larynx, pharynx, and guttural pouches
5. Ophthalmic structures
6. **Auricular structures**
7. Brain and nervous system
8. **Vascular anatomy**
9. Muscles
10. **Glandular structures – lymph and salivary**

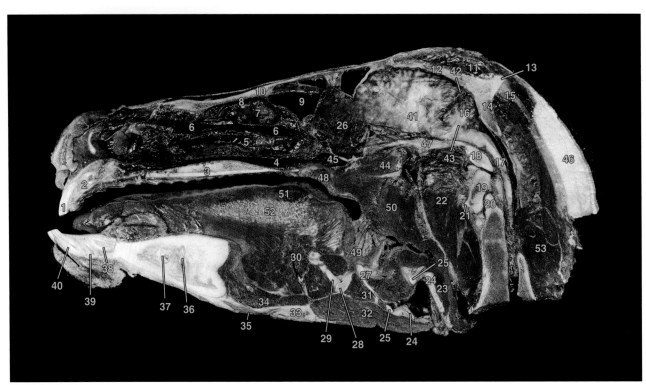

1 Tooth 201 (left superior central incisor)	21 **Ventral tubercle of the atlas**	39 Root of tooth 302 (left inferior intermediate incisor)
2 Root of tooth 202 (left superior intermediate incisor)	22 Longus capitis m.	
	23 Cricoarytenoideus dorsalis m.	40 Root and crown of tooth 301 (left inferior central incisor)
3 **Palantine process of the maxilla**	24 **Cricoid cartilage of the larynx**	
4 **Ventral meatus**	25 **Arytenoid cartilage of the larynx**	41 Thalamus
5 **Ventral concha**	26 **Ethmoid turbinates**	42 **Osseous tentorium cerebelli**
6 **Middle meatus**	27 **Epiglottic cartilage**	43 Cerebellar peduncle
7 **Dorsal concha**	28 **Basihyoid bone**	44 Tensor muscle of soft palate
8 **Dorsal meatus**	29 **Ceratohyoid bone**	45 **Sphenopalatine opening**
9 **Conchofrontal sinus**	30 Hyoglossus m.	46 **Nuchal adipose body**
10 **Nasal bone**	31 Thyrohyoideus m.	47 **Body of basisphenoid bone**
11 Temporalis m.	32 Sternohyoideus m. and omohyoideus m.	48 **Soft palate**
12 **Parietal bone**	33 **Mandibular lymph nodes**	49 **Palatine tonsil**
13 **Nuchal crest**	34 Geniohyoideus m.	50 Hyopharyngeus m.
14 **Squamous portion of the occipital bone**	35 Mylohyoideus m.	51 Intrinsic muscle of tongue (longitudinal fibers)
15 Nuchal ligament (funicular portion)	36 **Distal root of tooth 306 (left inferior second premolar)**	
16 Cerebellum		52 Intrinsic muscle of tongue (transverse fibers)
17 Spinal cord	37 **Mesial root of tooth 306 (left inferior second premolar)**	
18 **Basilar portion of the occipital bone**		53 Multifidus cervicis m.
19 **Ventral arch of the atlas**	38 **Root of tooth 303 (left inferior corner incisor)**	
20 **Dens of the axis**		

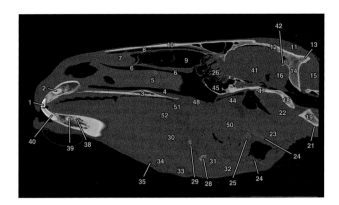

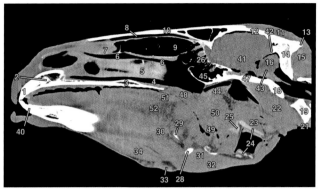

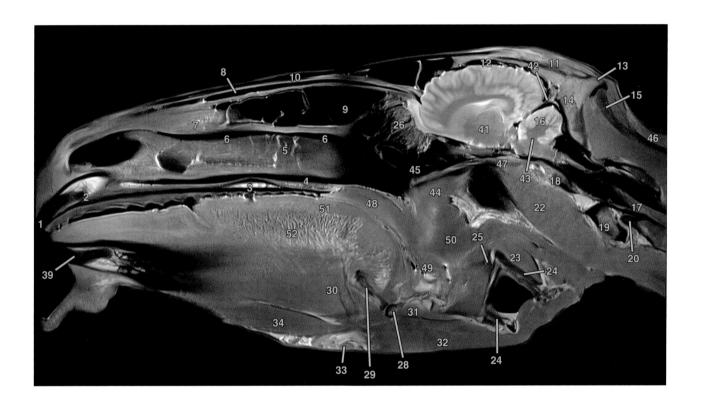

S7

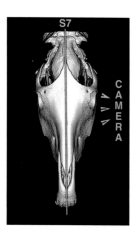

1. **Bones of the head**
2. **Oral and dental structures**
3. **Nasal and sinus structures**
4. Larynx, pharynx, and guttural pouches
5. **Ophthalmic structures**
6. **Auricular structures**
7. Brain and nervous system
8. **Vascular anatomy**
9. Muscles
10. **Glandular structures – lymph and salivary**

Brain structures covered separately

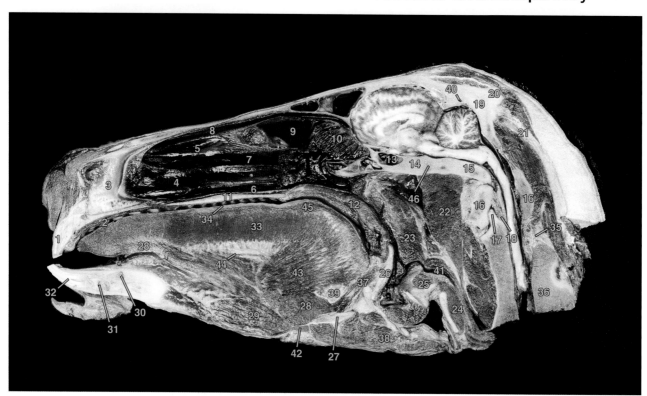

1 Tooth 201 (left superior central incisor)	18 Longitudinal ligament of the dens	33 Intrinsic muscle of tongue (perpendicular fibers)
2 Palatine rugae	19 **Occipital bone, squamous portion**	
3 Rostral extent of the nasal septum	20 **Nuchal crest**	34 Lingual mucosa
4 Ventral concha	21 Nuchal ligament (funicular portion)	35 Dorsal atlantoaxial ligament
5 Dorsal concha	22 Longus capitis m.	36 **Spinous process of C2 (axis)**
6 Ventral meatus	23 Hyopharyngeus m.	37 Hyoepiglotticus m.
7 Middle meatus	24 Cricoarytenoideus dorsalis m.	38 Sternohyoideus m.
8 Dorsal meatus	25 Arytenoid cartilage	39 Hyoideus transversus m.
9 Conchofrontal sinus	26 Epiglottis	40 **Transverse venous sinus**
10 Ethmoid turbinates	27 **Lingual process of basihyoid bone**	41 Esophageal lumen
11 Palatine process of the maxilla	28 Hyoglossus m.	42 Mylohyoideus m.
12 Soft palate	29 Geniohyoideus m.	43 Genioglossus m.
13 Sphenopalatine sinus	30 **Tooth 303 (left inferior corner incisor)**	44 **Deep lingual artery and vein**
14 **Basiphenoid bone**	31 **Tooth 302 (left inferior intermediate incisor)**	45 Intrinsic muscle of tongue (longitudinal fibers)
15 **Occipital bone, basilar part**		
16 **Atlas**	32 **Tooth 301 (left inferior central incisor)**	46 **Sphenooccipital synchondrosis**
17 **Dens of the axis**		

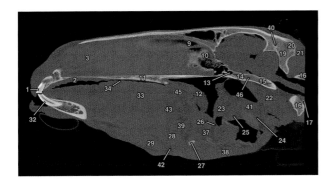

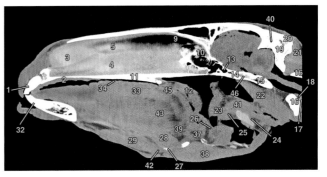

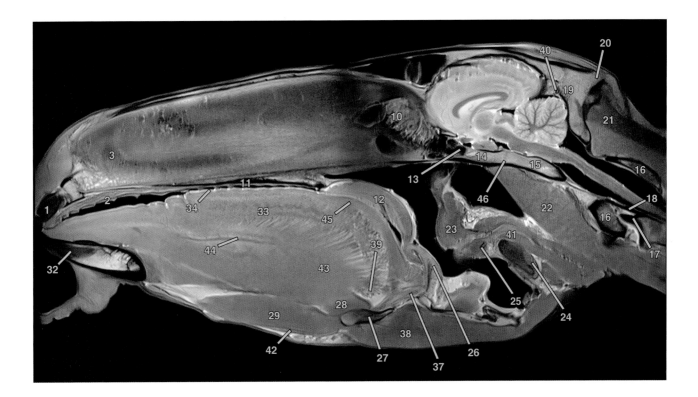

Brain sagittal close-up

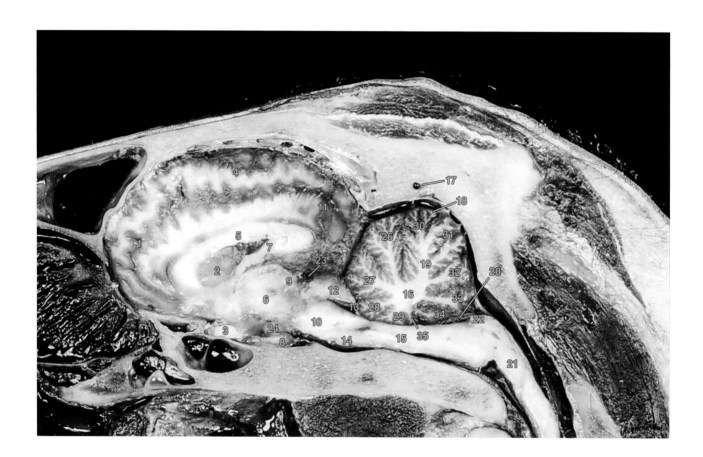

1 Frontal lobe
2 Lateral ventricle
3 Optic chiasm
4 Parietal lobe
5 Corpus callosum
6 Interthalamic adhesion
7 Hippocampus
8 Hypophysis (pituitary gland)
9 Third ventricle
10 Midbrain (tegmentum of mesencephalon)
11 Occipital lobe
12 Tectum of mesencephalon (roof of midbrain)

13 Mesencephalic aqueduct
14 Pons
15 Medulla oblongata
16 Central white matter (cerebellum)
17 **Transverse venous sinus**
18 Cerebellar cortex
19 Arbor vitae (branching white matter, "tree of life")
20 Choroid plexus (fourth ventricle)
21 Spinal cord
22 Obex
23 Pineal gland
24 Mamillary body

25 Central canal (not seen on cadaver image)
26 Pars caudalis
27 Pars rostralis
28 Lobulus centralis
29 Lingula cerebelli
30 Declive
31 Folium vermis
32 Tuber vermis
33 Pyramis (vermis)
34 Uvula (vermis)
35 Nodulus

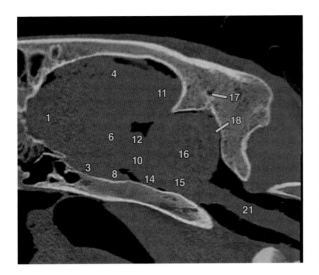

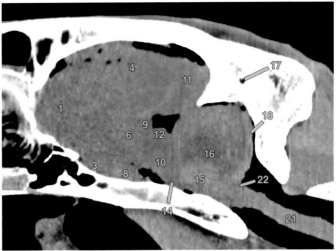

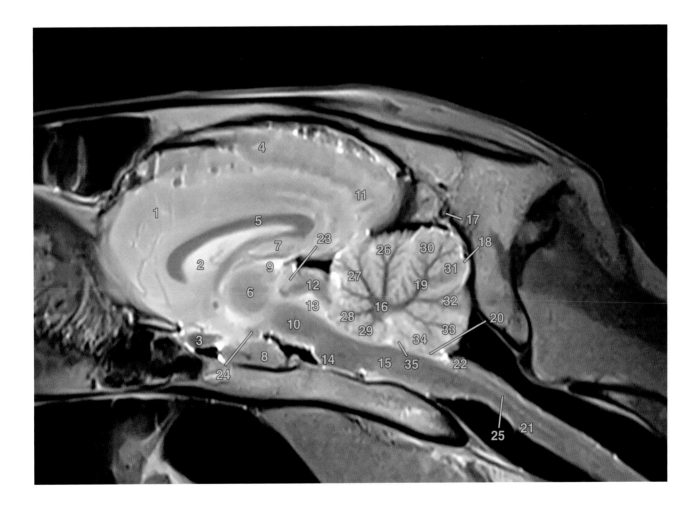

S8

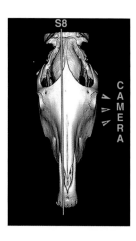

1. **Bones of the head**
2. **Oral and dental structures**
3. **Nasal and sinus structures**
4. Larynx, pharynx, and guttural pouches
5. **Ophthalmic structures**
6. **Auricular structures**
7. Brain and nervous system
8. **Vascular anatomy**
9. Muscles
10. **Glandular structures – lymph and salivary**

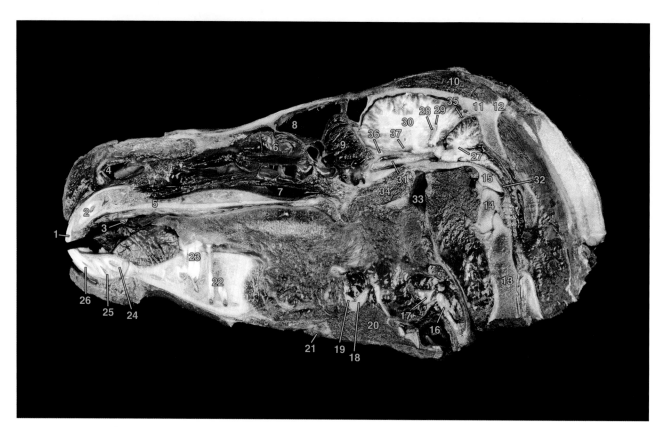

1 Tooth 102 (right superior intermediate incisor)	17 Arytenoid cartilage	29 Lateral ventricle (caudal aspect)
2 Tooth 103 (right superior corner incisor)	**18 Thyrohyoid bone**	30 Internal capsule
3 Tooth 104 (right superior canine tooth)	**19 Ceratohyoid bone**	31 Maxillary n. (branch of trigeminal n. in foramen rotundum)
4 Nasal diverticulum	20 Omohyoideus and thyrohyoideus mm.	
5 Palatine process of the maxilla	**21 Mandibular lymph node**	**32 Basilar a.**
6 Dorsal nasal concha	22 Root of tooth 407 (right inferior third premolar)	33 Auditory diverticulum (guttural pouch), medial compartment
7 Ventral meatus	23 Root of tooth 406 (right inferior second premolar)	34 Lateral pterygoid m.
8 Conchofrontal sinus		**35 Osseous tentorium cerebelli**
9 Ethmoidal labyrinth	24 Root of tooth 404 (root of the right inferior canine tooth)	36 Optic n. (in optic canal) (not seen on cadaver image)
10 Temporalis m.	25 Root of tooth 403 (root of the right inferior corner incisor)	37 Optic tract (to meet lateral geniculate nucleus) (not seen on cadaver image)
11 Occipital bone	26 Tooth 402 (right inferior intermediate incisor)	
12 Nuchal crest		38 Root of tooth 408 (right inferior fourth premolar) (not seen on cadaver image)
13 Axis	27 Cerebellar peduncle	
14 Atlas	28 Hippocampus	**39 Stylohyoid bone (not seen on cadaver image)**
15 Occipital condyle (ventral surface)		
16 Cricoid cartilage		

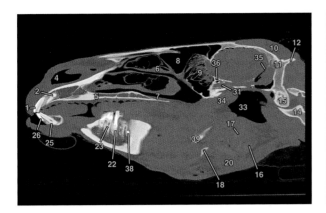

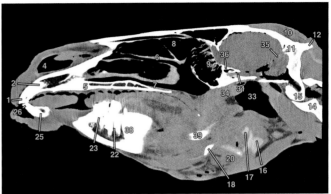

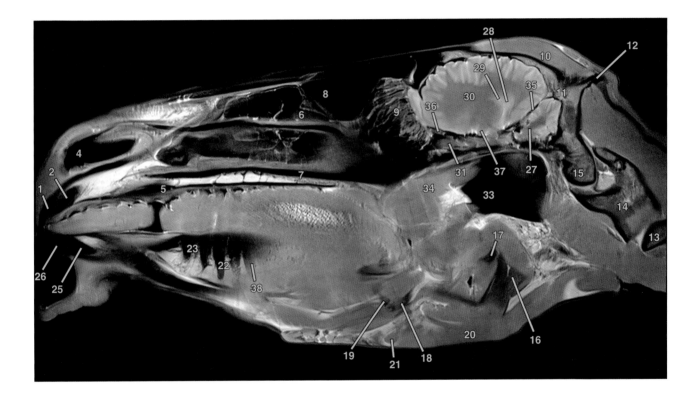

S9

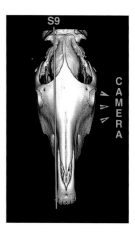

1. Bones of the head
2. Oral and dental structures
3. Nasal and sinus structures
4. Larynx, pharynx, and guttural pouches
5. Ophthalmic structures
6. Auricular structures
7. Brain and nervous system
8. Vascular anatomy
9. Muscles
10. Glandular structures – lymph and salivary

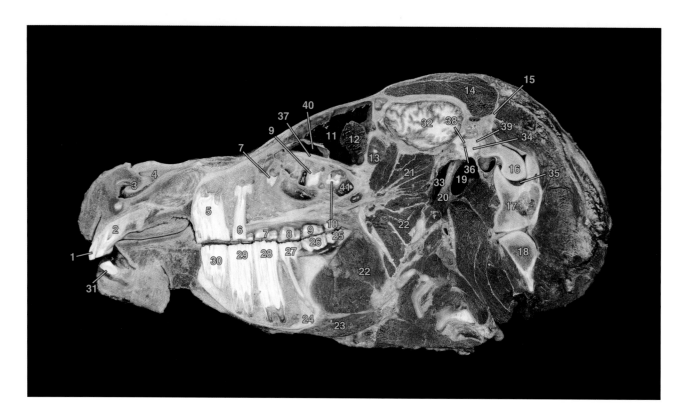

1 Tooth number 102 (right superior intermediate incisor)	14 Temporalis m.	29 Tooth 407 (right inferior third premolar)
2 Tooth number 103 (right superior corner incisor)	15 Nuchal crest	30 Tooth 406 (right inferior second premolar)
3 Alar fold	16 Occipital condyle	31 Tooth 403 (right inferior corner incisor)
4 Nasal diverticulum	17 Atlas	32 Temporal lobe
5 Tooth 106 (right superior second premolar)	18 Axis	33 Auditory diverticulum (guttural pouch), lateral compartment
6 Tooth 107 (right superior third premolar)	19 Auditory diverticulum (guttural pouch), medial compartment	
7 Tooth 108 (right superior fourth premolar)	20 Stylohyoid bone	34 Petrosal part of temporal bone
8 Tooth 109 (right superior first molar)	21 Lateral pterygoid m.	35 Atlanto-occipital joint
9 Tooth 110 (right superior second molar)	22 Medial pterygoid m.	36 Cochlea
10 Tooth 111 (right superior third molar)	23 Digastricus m., rostral belly	37 Infraorbital canal/n.
11 Conchofrontal sinus	24 Mandible	38 Facial nerve (cranial n.VII)
12 Ethmoidal labyrinth	25 Tooth 411 (right inferior third molar)	39 Semi-circular canal
13 Retrobulbar mm. and optic n.	26 Tooth 410 (right inferior second molar)	40 Ventral conchal sinus
	27 Tooth 409 (right inferior first molar)	41 Caudal maxillary sinus
	28 Tooth 408 (right inferior fourth premolar)	

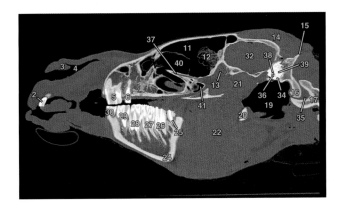

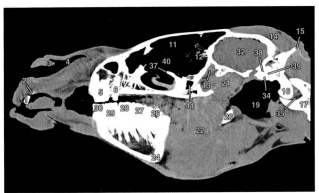

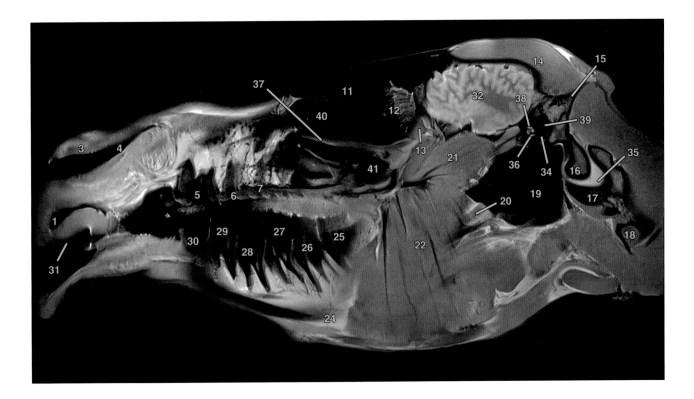

S10

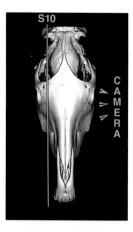

1. **Bones of the head**
2. Oral and dental structures
3. **Nasal and sinus structures**
4. Larynx, pharynx, and guttural pouches
5. **Ophthalmic structures**
6. **Auricular structures**
7. Brain and nervous system
8. **Vascular anatomy**
9. Muscles
10. **Glandular structures – lymph and salivary**

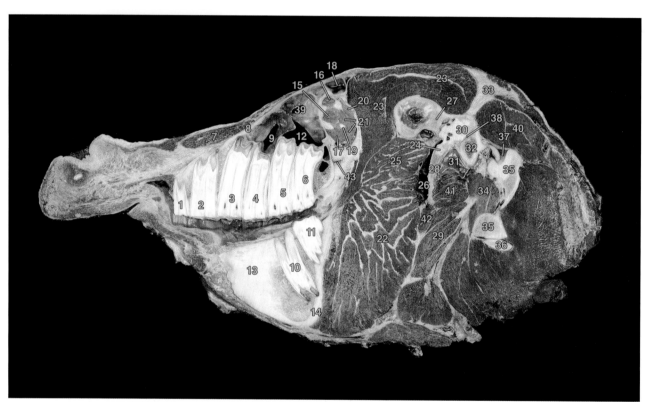

1 Tooth 106 (right superior second premolar)	15 Medial rectus m.	31 Auditory diverticulum (guttural pouch), medial compartment (dorsolateral wall)
2 Tooth 107 (right superior third premolar)	16 Dorsal oblique m.	32 Occipital bone (lateral aspect – start of paracondyloid process)
3 Tooth 108 (right superior fourth premolar)	17 Ventral rectus m.	
	18 Frontal sinus	33 Auricular adipose body
4 Tooth 109 (right superior first molar)	19 Optic n.	34 Rectus capitis ventralis m.
5 Tooth 110 (right superior second molar)	20 Dorsal rectus m.	35 Atlas
6 Tooth 111 (right upper third molar)	21 Retractor bulbi m.	36 Axis
7 Levator labii superioris m.	22 Medial pterygoid m.	37 Atlanto-occipital joint (lateral aspect)
8 Maxilla	23 Temporalis m.	38 Occipitomastoid suture
9 Maxillary sinus, rostral portion	24 Tympanohyoideum	39 Conchofrontal sinus
10 Tooth 410 (right inferior second molar)	25 Lateral pterygoid m.	40 Obliquus capitis cranialis m.
11 Tooth 411 (right inferior third molar)	26 Auditory diverticulum (guttural pouch), lateral compartment	41 Occipitohyoid m.
12 Maxillary sinus, caudal portion	27 Squamous part of the temporal bone	42 Stylohyoid m.
13 Lateral cortex of the body of the mandible	28 Stylohyoid bone	43 Deep facial vein
	29 Digastricus m. (caudal portion)	
14 Medial cortex of the body of the mandible	30 Petrosal part of the temporal bone	

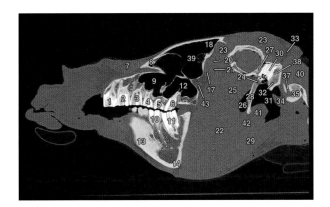

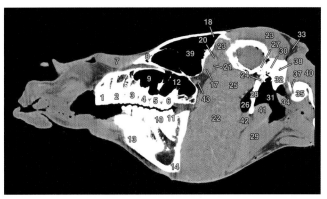

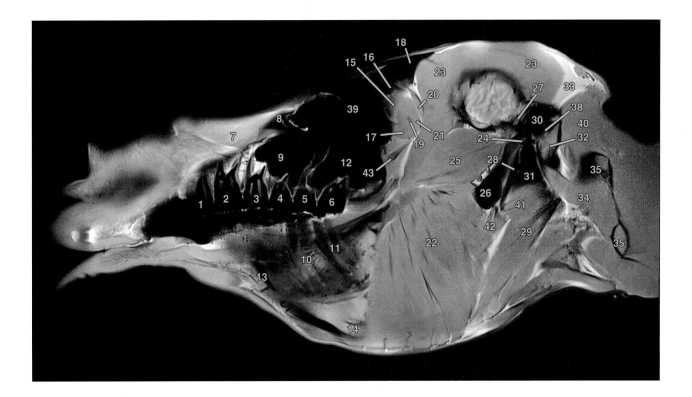

S11

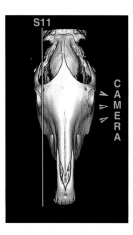

1. **Bones of the head**
2. **Oral and dental structures**
3. **Nasal and sinus structures**
4. Larynx, pharynx, and guttural pouches
5. **Ophthalmic structures**
6. **Auricular structures**
7. Brain and nervous system
8. **Vascular anatomy**
9. Muscles
10. **Glandular structures – lymph and salivary**

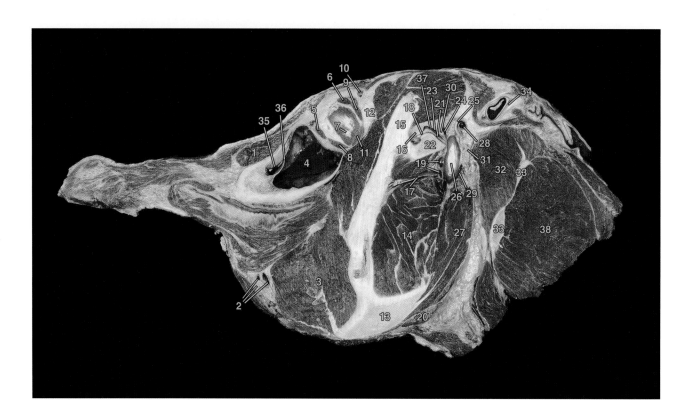

1 Levator labii superioris m.	17 Maxillary v.	28 External auditory meatus
2 Facial a. and v. and parotid duct	18 Articular disk of the temporomandibular joint	29 Caudal auricular v.
3 Masseter m.		30 Retroarticular process
4 Caudal maxillary sinus	19 Superficial temporal vein	31 Parotid salivary gland
5 Ventral oblique m.	20 Mandibular salivary gland	32 Obliquus capitis cranialis m.
6 Dorsal oblique m.	21 Caudal fibrous expansion of the articular disk of the temporomandibular joint	33 Transverse process (wing) of the atlas
7 Optic n.		34 Auricular cartilage
8 Ventral rectus m.		35 Rostral maxillary sinus
9 Dorsal rectus m.	22 Condylar process of the mandible	36 Maxillary sinus septum
10 Lateral aspect of frontal sinus	23 Mandibular fossa of the temporal bone	37 Articular tuberculum
11 Retractor bulbi m.	24 Temporal venous sinus	38 Obliquus capitis caudalis m.
12 Orbital adipose body	25 Annular cartilage	
13 Angle of the mandible	26 Auditory diverticulum (guttural pouch) (lateral-most aspect of the lateral compartment)	
14 Medial pterygoid m.		
15 Coronoid process of the mandible		
16 Articular tubercle of the temporal bone	27 Digastricus m.	

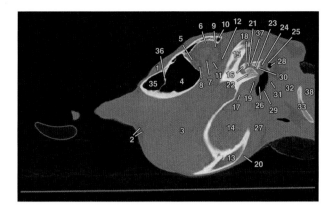

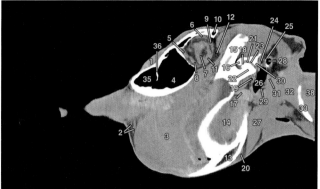

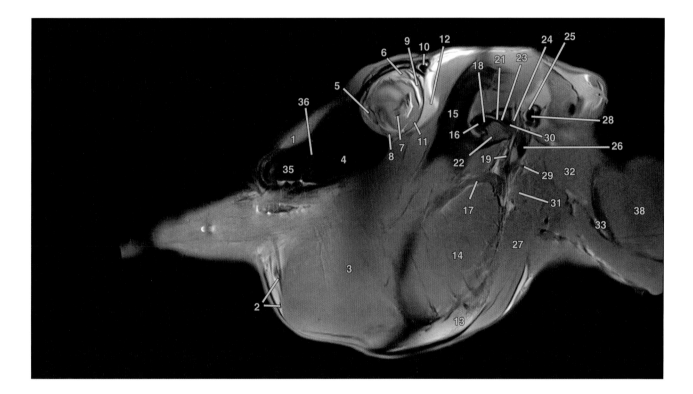

S12

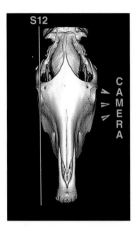

1. **Bones of the head**
2. Oral and dental structures
3. **Nasal and sinus structures**
4. Larynx, pharynx, and guttural pouches
5. Ophthalmic structures
6. **Auricular structures**
7. Brain and nervous system
8. **Vascular anatomy**
9. Muscles
10. **Glandular structures – lymph and salivary**

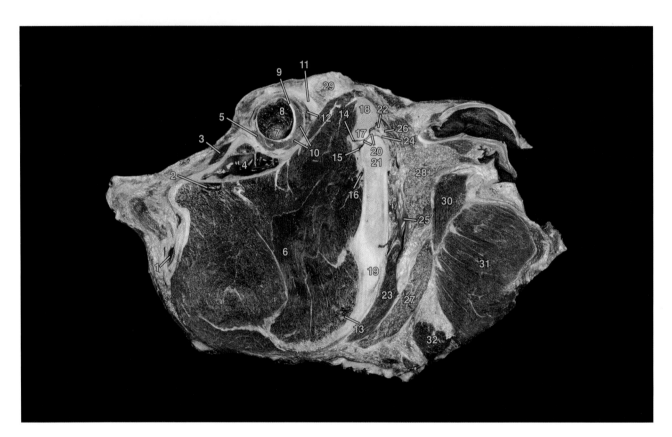

1 Facial v.	15 Rostral compartment of the ventral synovial pouch of the temporomandibular joint	25 Maxillary v.
2 Deep facial v.		26 Articular capsule of the temporomandibular joint
3 Levator labii superioris m.		27 Mandibular salivary gland
4 Caudal maxillary sinus	16 Transverse facial v.	28 Parotid salivary gland
5 Ventral rectus m.	17 Articular tubercle	29 Adipose body of temporal fossa
6 Masseter m.	18 Zygomatic process of the temporal bone	30 Cranial obliquus capitis m.
7 Lens	19 Caudal border of the mandible	31 Caudal obliquus capitis m.
8 Vitreous	20 Articular disk of the temporomandibular joint	32 Longus capitis m.
9 Sclera	21 Condylar process of the mandible	
10 Retractor bulbi m.	22 Caudal compartment of the dorsal synovial pouch of the temporomandibular joint	
11 Frontal bone		
12 Lacrimal gland	23 Digastricus m.	
13 Ventral masseteric v.	24 Caudal fibrous expansion of the articular disk	
14 Rostral compartment of the dorsal synovial pouch of the temporomandibular joint		

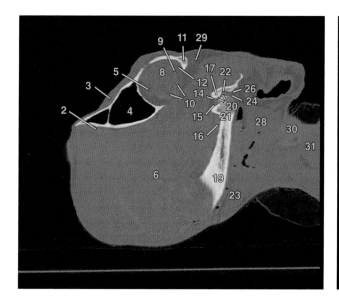

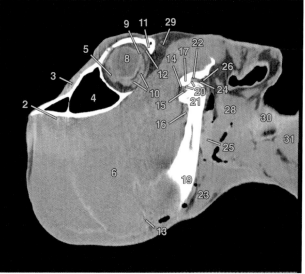

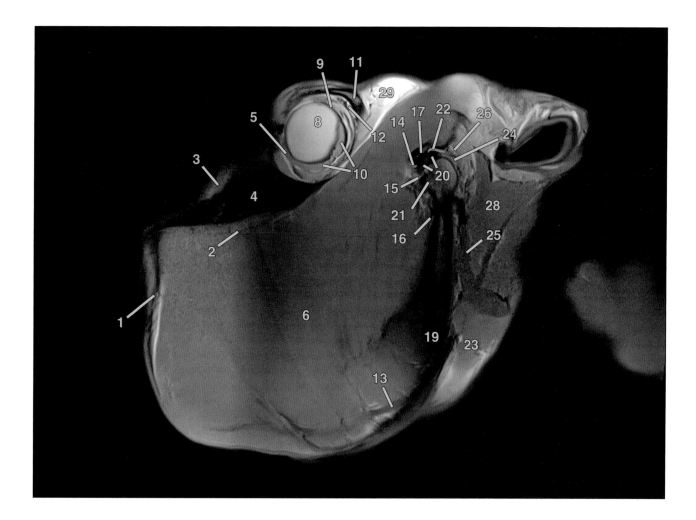

S13

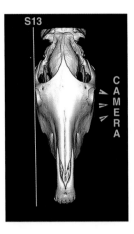

1. **Bones of the head**
2. Oral and dental structures
3. **Nasal and sinus structures**
4. Larynx, pharynx, and guttural pouches
5. Ophthalmic structures
6. **Auricular structures**
7. Brain and nervous system
8. **Vascular anatomy**
9. Muscles
10. **Glandular structures – lymph and salivary**

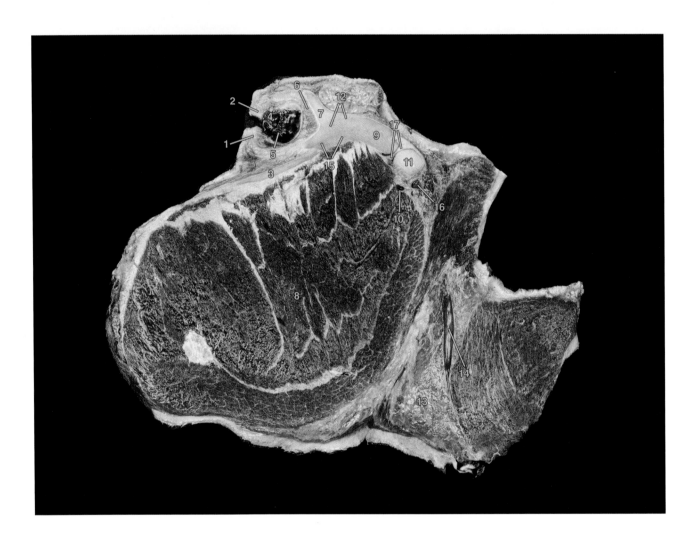

1 Palpebra inferior (lower eyelid)	8 Masseter m.	14 Maxillary v.
2 Palpebra superior (upper eyelid	9 Temporal bone	15 Temporozygomatic suture
3 Facial crest (zygomatic bone)	10 Transverse facial vein	16 Superficial temporal vein
4 Anterior chamber of the eye	11 Condylar process of the mandible	17 Articular disk of the temporomandibular
5 Iris	(lateral aspect)	joint
6 Lacrimal gland	12 Temporofrontal suture	18 Lens (cannot see on cadaver)
7 Zygomatic process of the frontal bone	13 Parotid salivary gland (ventral aspect)	

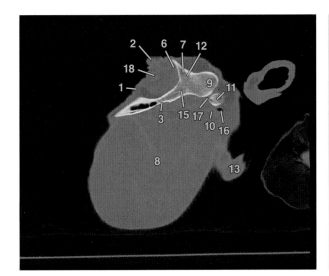

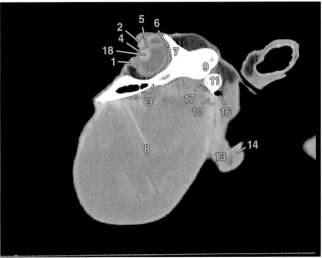

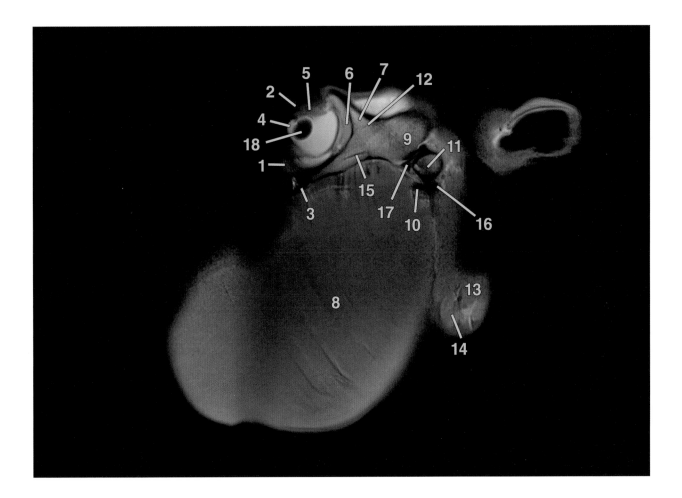

CHAPTER 4

Clinical and Surgical Anatomy of the Equine Head: Dorsal Sections

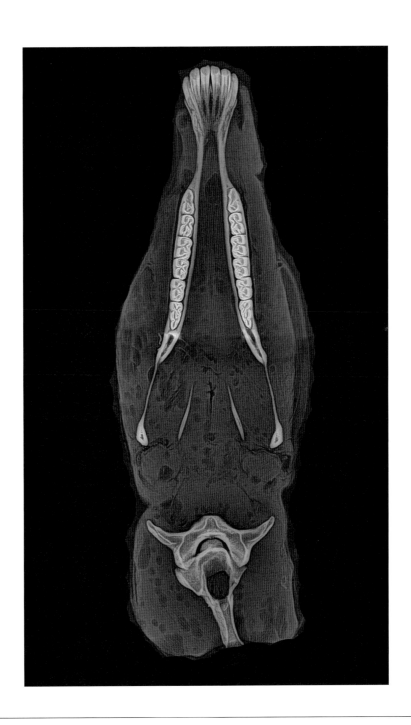

Atlas of Clinical Imaging and Anatomy of the Equine Head, First Edition. Larry Kimberlin, Alex zur Linden and Lynn Ruoff.
© 2017 John Wiley & Sons, Inc. Published 2017 by John Wiley & Sons, Inc.

D1

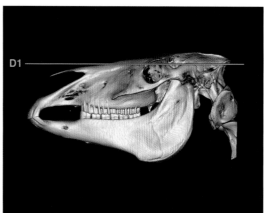

1. **Bones of the head**
2. Oral and dental structures
3. **Nasal and sinus structures**
4. Larynx, pharynx, and guttural pouches
5. **Ophthalmic structures**
6. **Auricular structures**
7. Brain and nervous system
8. **Vascular anatomy**
9. Muscles
10. **Glandular structures – lymph and salivary**

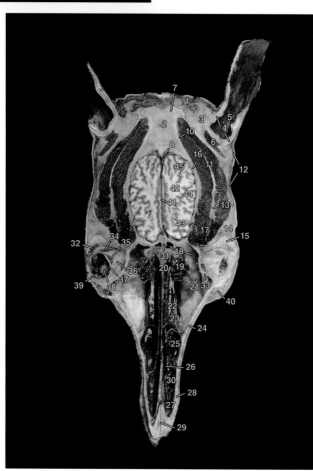

1 Caudal auricular mm.
2 Occipital bone
3 Auricular adipose body
4 Auricular cartilage
5 External ear canal
6 Rostral auricular mm.
7 Nuchal crest
8 Sagittal venous sinus
9 Transverse venous sinus (not seen on cadaver)
10 Rostral deep temporal a. and v.
11 Temporalis m.
12 Parotidoauricularis m.
13 Coronoid process of the mandible
14 Orbital adipose body
15 Zygomatic process of the frontal bone

16 Parietal bone
17 Frontal bone
18 Frontal sinus
19 Ethmoidal labyrinth
20 Perpendicular plate of the ethmoid bone
21 Conchofrontal sinus
22 Dorsal nasal conchae
23 Nasal septum (cartilaginous portion)
24 Maxilla
25 Dorsal conchal sinus
26 Common nasal meatus
27 Dorsal conchal fold
28 Incisive bone
29 Internasal suture
30 Dorsal conchal bulla
31 Septum of frontal sinus

32 Lacrimal gland
33 Lacrimal bone
34 Lateral rectus m.
35 Retractor bulbi m.
36 Intraperiorbital adipose body
37 Sclera
38 Lens
39 Palpebra superioris
40 Orbicularis oculi m.
41 Longitudinal fissure of the cerebrum
42 Cerebral white matter
43 Frontal lobe
44 Parietal lobe
45 Occipital lobe

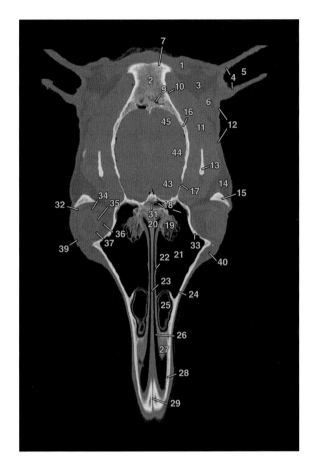

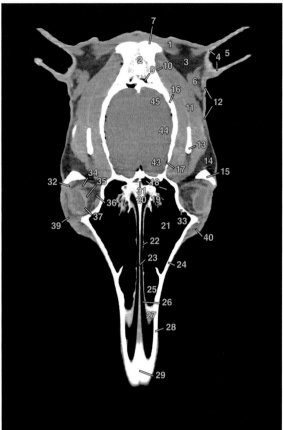

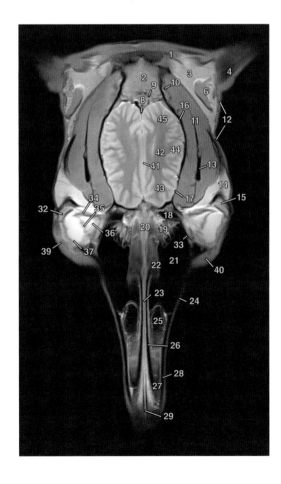

D2

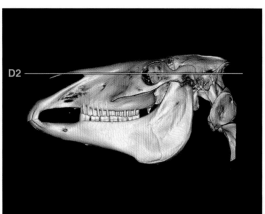

1. Bones of the head
2. Oral and dental structures
3. Nasal and sinus structures
4. Larynx, pharynx, and guttural pouches
5. Ophthalmic structures
6. Auricular structures
7. Brain and nervous system
8. Vascular anatomy
9. Muscles
10. Glandular structures – lymph and salivary

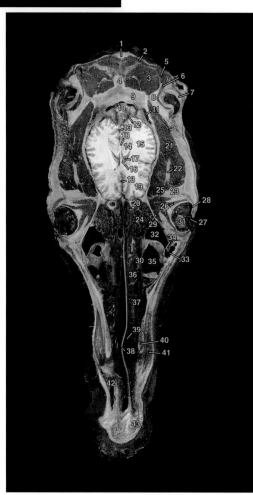

1 Nuchal ligament, funicular portion	15 White matter of cerebrum	30 Dorsal nasal concha
2 Cervicoauricularis superficialis m.	16 Lateral ventricle	31 Lens
3 Obliquus capitis cranialis m.	17 Choroid plexus (in lateral ventricle)	32 Conchofrontal sinus
4 External occipital protuberance	18 Corpus callosum	33 Caudal maxillary sinus
5 Cervicoauricularis profundus m.	19 Frontal lobe of the cerebrum	34 Frontomaxillary opening
6 Cervocoauricularis medialis m.	20 Olfactory lobe and recess	35 Ventral conchal sinus
7 Auricular cartilage	21 Temporalis m.	36 Conchofrontal opening
8 Auricular adipose body	22 Coronoid process of the mandible	37 Dorsal conchal sinus
9 Occipital bone	23 Ophthalmic adipose body	38 Nasal septum (cartilaginous portion)
10 Cerebellum (dorsal aspect)	24 Ethmoidal labyrinth	39 Common nasal meatus
11 Transverse sinus	25 Lateral rectus m.	40 Incisive bone
12 Tentorium cerebelli	26 Retractor bulbi m.	41 Levator labii superioris m.
13 Falx cerebri (within longitudinal fissure)	27 Iris	42 Nasal diverticulum
14 Hippocampus	28 Sclera	43 Dilator nasal apicalis m.
	29 Medial rectus m.	

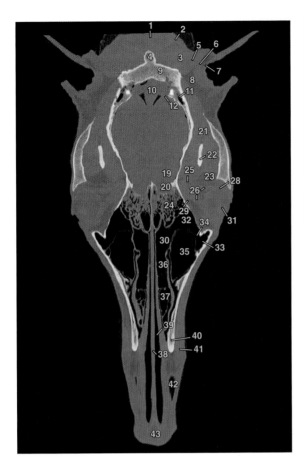

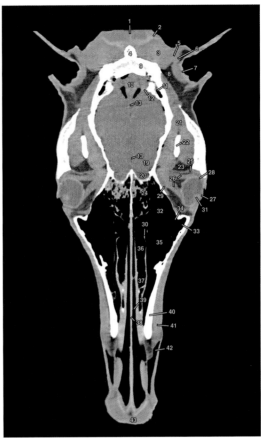

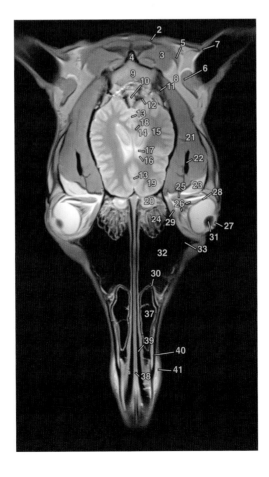

D3

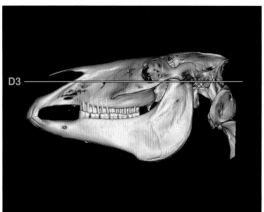

1. **Bones of the head**
2. Oral and dental structures
3. **Nasal and sinus structures**
4. Larynx, pharynx, and guttural pouches
5. **Ophthalmic structures**
6. **Auricular structures**
7. Brain and nervous system
8. **Vascular anatomy**
9. Muscles
10. **Glandular structures – lymph and salivary**

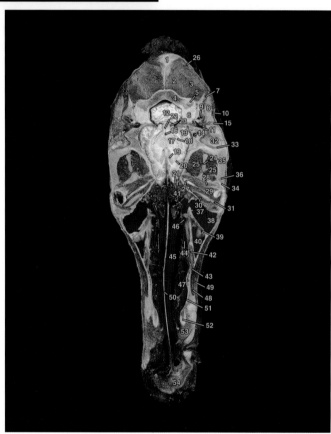

1 Nuchal ligament, funicular portion	19 Caudate nucleus	38 Caudal maxillary sinus
2 Rectus capitis dorsalis m.	20 Internal capsule	39 Maxillary sinus septum
3 Obliquus capitis cranialis m.	21 Cribriform plate	40 Rostral maxillary sinus
4 Occipital bone, squamous portion	22 Mesencephalic aqueduct	41 Ethmoidal labyrinth
5 Occipitomastoid suture	23 Rostral colliculus	42 Infraorbital canal (infraorbital n., a., v.)
6 Temporal bone (petrous part)	24 Coronoid process of the mandible	43 Infraorbital foramen
7 Cervicoauricularis m.	25 Masseter m.	44 Ventral conchal sinus
8 Auricular fat body	26 Semispinalis capitis m.	45 Common meatus
9 External ear canal	27 Optic n.	46 Conchomaxillary opening
10 Parotidoauricularis m.	28 Lateral rectus m.	47 Ventral conchal bulla
11 Temporal venous sinus	29 Retractor bulbi m.	48 Levator labii superioris m.
12 Cerebellum	30 Medial rectus m.	49 Levator nasolabialis m.
13 Caudal pole of cerebral hemisphere (occipital lobe)	31 Ventral oblique m.	50 Nasal septum
14 Ventral petrous venous sinus	32 Condyloid process of the mandible	51 Maxilla
15 Parotid salivary gland	33 Articular disk	52 Incisive bone
16 Third ventricle	34 Temporal process of the zygomatic bone	53 Dorsal part of lateral nasal m.
17 Thalamus	35 Zygomatic process of the temporal bone	54 Dilator naris apicalis m.
18 Hippocampus	36 Temporozygomatic suture	
	37 Frontomaxillary opening	

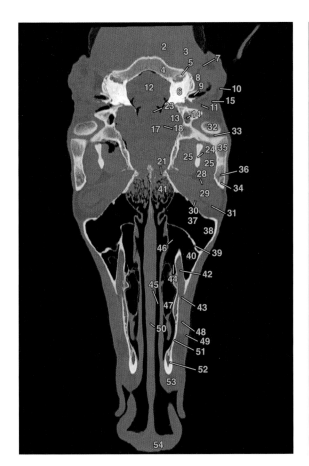

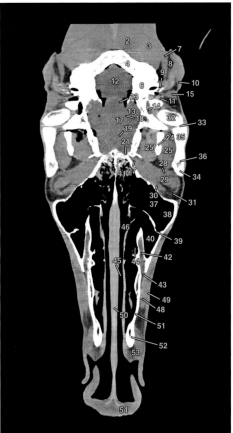

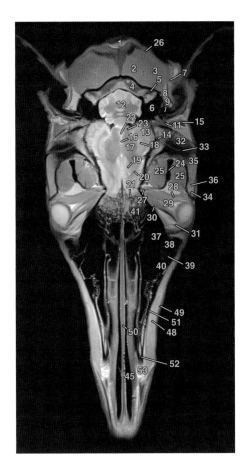

D4

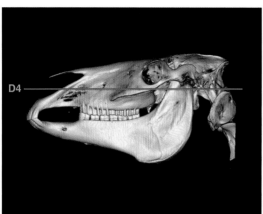

1. Bones of the head
2. Oral and dental structures
3. Nasal and sinus structures
4. Larynx, pharynx, and guttural pouches
5. Ophthalmic structures
6. Auricular structures
7. Brain and nervous system
8. Vascular anatomy
9. Muscles
10. Glandular structures – lymph and salivary

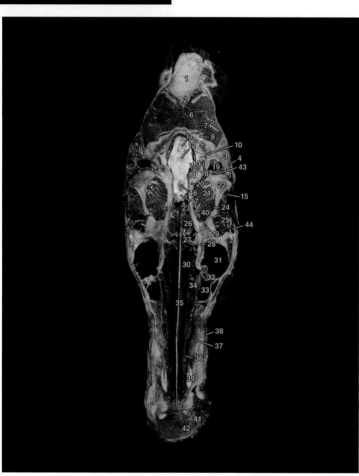

1 Nuchal adipose body
2 Nuchal ligament, funicular portion
3 Parotid salivary gland
4 Parotidoauricularis m.
5 Obliquus capitis cranialis m.
6 Rectus capitis dorsalis m.
7 Cranial articular surface of the atlas
8 Occipital condyle
9 Occipital bone
10 Occipitomastoid suture
11 Cerebellar vermis
12 Cerebellar lingula
13 Facial n.
14 Caudal cerebellar peduncle
15 Masseteric v. and a.
16 Pituitary gland

17 Optic chiasm
18 Temporal bone, tympanic portion
19 Auditory diverticulum (guttural pouch), lateral compartment
20 Trigeminal n.
21 Lateral pterygoid m.
22 Condylar (condyloid) process of the mandible
23 Sphenoidal sinus
24 Temporalis profunda v.
25 Masseter m.
26 Ethmoidal labyrinth
27 Lacrimal bone
28 Infraorbital n.
29 Deep facial v.
30 Common nasal meatus

31 Maxillary sinus, caudal compartment
32 Maxillary sinus septum
33 Maxillary sinus, rostral compartment
34 Ventral concha
35 Nasal septum
36 Ventral conchal bulla
37 Maxillary bone
38 Levator nasolabialis m.
39 Incisive bone
40 Temporalis m.
41 Cornu of alar cartilage
42 Dilator naris apicalis m.
43 Temporomandibular joint branch of the superficial temporal a.
44 Transverse facial v. sinus

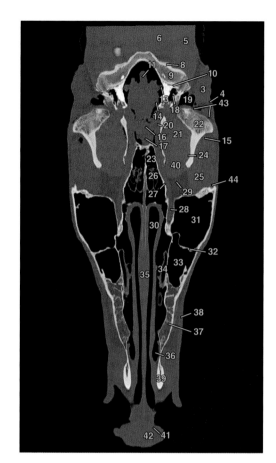
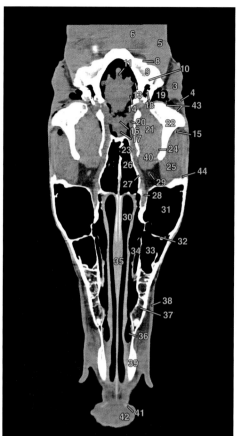
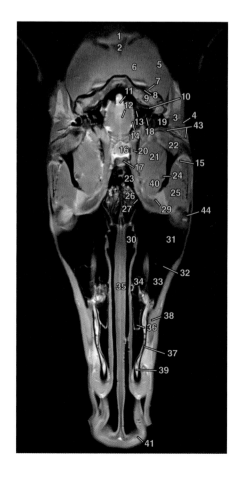

D5

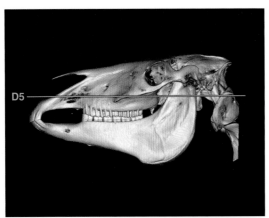

1. **Bones of the head**
2. Oral and dental structures
3. **Nasal and sinus structures**
4. Larynx, pharynx, and guttural pouches
5. **Ophthalmic structures**
6. **Auricular structures**
7. Brain and nervous system
8. **Vascular anatomy**
9. Muscles
10. **Glandular structures – lymph and salivary**

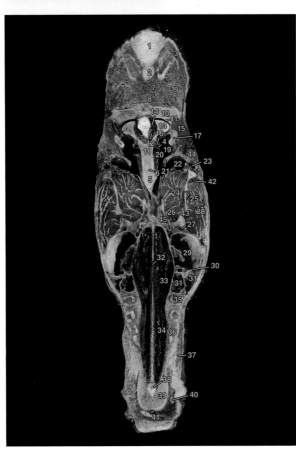

1 Nuchal adipose body	18 Occipital bone, basilar portion	33 Ventral concha
2 Nuchal ligament, funicular portion	19 Auditory diverticulum (guttural pouch), medial compartment	34 Common nasal meatus
3 Splenius m.		35 Reserve crown, tooth 208 (left superior fourth premolar)
4 Vagus n. (CN 10)	20 Longus capitis m.	
5 Basisphenoid bone	21 Stylohyoid bone	36 Reserve crown, tooth 206 (left superior second premolar)
6 Sphenooccipital synchondrosis	22 Auditory diverticulum (guttural pouch), lateral compartment	
7 Rectus capitis dorsalis major m.		37 Levator nasolabialis m.
8 Rectus capitis dorsalis minor m.	23 Superficial temporalis v.	38 Vomeronasal organ
9 Obliquus capitis caudalis m.	24 Lateral pterygoid m.	39 Incisive bone
10 Atlas	25 Ramus of the mandible	40 Cornu of the alar cartilage
11 Atlantooccipital joint	26 Infraorbital a.	41 Dilator naris apicalis m.
12 Dura mater	27 Deep facial v.	42 Masseteric v. and a.
13 Occipital condyle	28 Masseter m.	43 Temporalis profunda v.
14 Arachnoid and subarachnoid space	29 Caudal maxillary sinus	44 Parotid salivary gland
15 Obliquus capitis cranialis m.	30 Septum of the maxillary sinus	45 Sphenoidal sinus (ventral aspect)
16 Internal carotid a.	31 Rostral maxillary sinus	
17 Paracondylar process	32 Nasal septum	

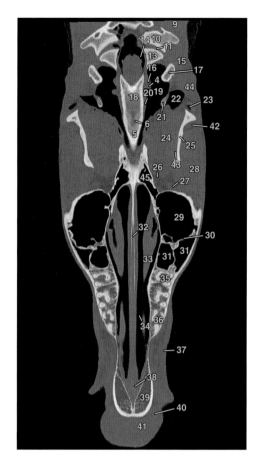

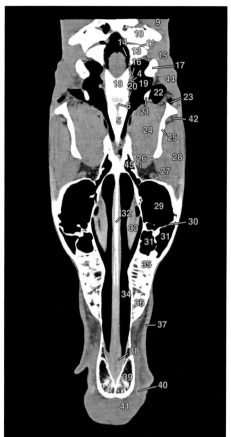

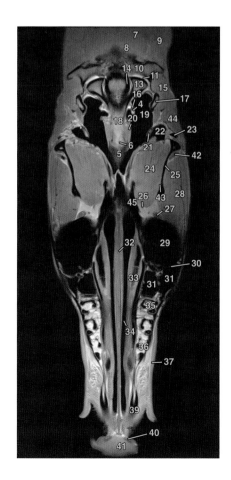

D6

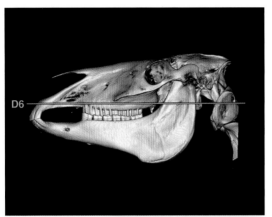

1. Bones of the head
2. Oral and dental structures
3. Nasal and sinus structures
4. Larynx, pharynx, and guttural pouches
5. Ophthalmic structures
6. Auricular structures
7. Brain and nervous system
8. Vascular anatomy
9. Muscles
10. Glandular structures – lymph and salivary

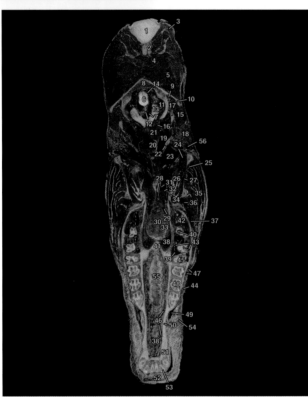

1 Nuchal adipose body
2 Nuchal ligament, funicular portion
3 Splenius m.
4 Rectus capitis dorsalis m.
5 Obliquus capitis caudalis m.
6 Cervical spinal cord
7 Ventral internal vertebral venous plexus
8 Dorsal arch of the atlas
9 Vertebral artery and vein
10 Wing of the atlas
11 Atlantooccipital joint
12 Dura mater
13 Occipital condyle
14 Arachnoid and subarachnoid space
15 Obliquus capitis cranialis m.
16 Internal carotid a., vagus n., accessory n., sympathetic trunk
17 Paracondylar process
18 Parotid salivary gland
19 Auditory diverticulum (guttural pouch), medial compartment
20 Longus capitis m.

21 Ventral rectus capitis m.
22 Stylohyoid bone
23 Auditory diverticulum (guttural pouch), lateral compartment
24 Maxillary v.
25 Masseteric v. and a.
26 Medial pterygoid m.
27 Ramus of the mandible
28 Nasopharynx
29 Pharyngeal mm.
30 Palatinus m.
31 Levator m. of the soft palate
32 Tensor m. of the soft palate
33 Palatopharyngeus m.
34 Pterygoid bone
35 Masseter m.
36 Buccal venous sinus
37 Transverse facial venous sinus
38 Ventral nasal venous plexus
39 Rostral maxillary sinus
40 Reserve crown of tooth 211 (left fourth superior molar)

41 Caudal border of horizontal portion of the palatine bone
42 Caudal maxillary sinus
43 Septum of the maxillary sinus
44 Buccinator m.
45 Reserve crown of tooth 209 (left superior first molar)
46 Greater palatine a.
47 Facial v. and a.
48 Reserve crown of tooth 207 (left superior third premolar)
49 Oral cavity vestibule
50 Maxilla
51 Incisive bone
52 Orbicularis oris m.
53 Reserve crown tooth 202 (left superior middle incisor)
54 Caninus m.
55 Palatine bone (hard palate)
56 Superficial temporal v.

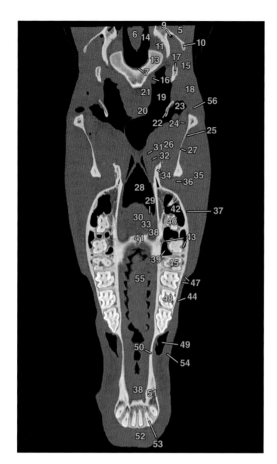

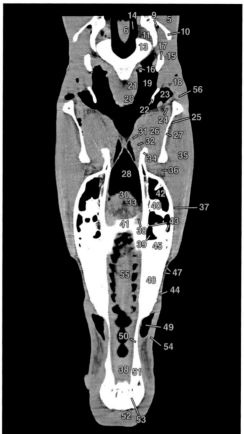

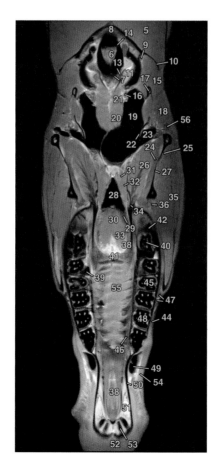

D7

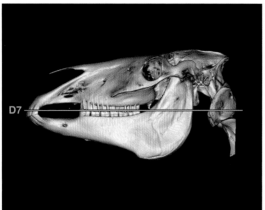

1. **Bones of the head**
2. Oral and dental structures
3. **Nasal and sinus structures**
4. Larynx, pharynx, and guttural pouches
5. **Ophthalmic structures**
6. **Auricular structures**
7. Brain and nervous system
8. **Vascular anatomy**
9. Muscles
10. **Glandular structures – lymph and salivary**

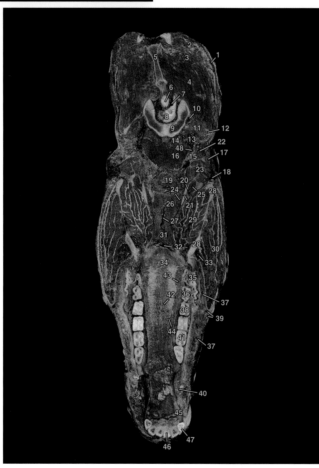

1 Splenius m.	18 **Maxillary v.**	35 **Tooth 211 (left superior third molar)**
2 Rhomboideus m.	19 **Esophagus**	36 **Tooth 310 (left inferior second molar)**
3 Semispinalis capitis m.	20 **External carotid a.**	37 Buccinator m.
4 Obliquus capitis caudalis m.	21 **Stylohyoid bone**	38 **Tooth 309 (left inferior first molar)**
5 **Spinous process of the axis**	22 **Mandibular salivary gland**	39 **Facial a. and v.**
6 Spinal cord	23 Digastricus m.	40 **Buccal salivary glands**
7 **Ventral vertebral vv.**	24 Stylopharyngeal m.	41 **Tooth 307 (left inferior second premolar)**
8 **Body of the axis (C2)**	25 Stylohyoideus m.	42 Genioglossus m.
9 **Ventral arch of the atlas (C1)**	26 Pharyngeal mm.	43 Styloglossus m.
10 **Vertebral a.**	27 **Nasopharynx (collapsed)**	44 Hyoglossus m.
11 Obliquus capitis cranialis m.	28 **Ramus of the mandible**	45 **Mandible**
12 **Wing of the atlas**	29 Medial pterygoid m.	46 **Pulp cavity, tooth 301 (left inferior central incisor)**
13 **Occipital v.**	30 Masseter m.	
14 Ventral rectus capitis m.	31 **Soft palate**	47 **Tooth 303 (left inferior corner incisor)**
15 **Internal carotid a.**	32 Oropharynx	48 **Occipital a.**
16 Longus capitis m.	33 **Buccal venous sinus**	
17 **Parotid salivary gland**	34 **Intrinsic muscles of the tongue**	

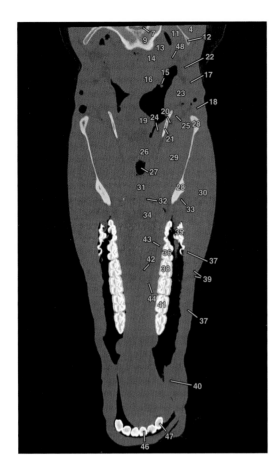

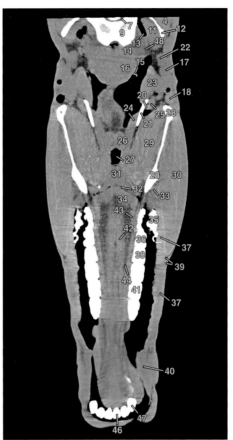

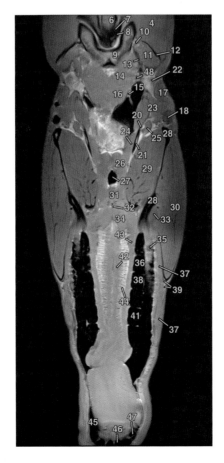

D8

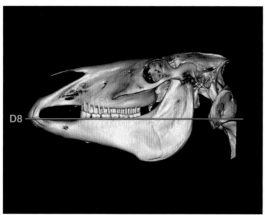

1. **Bones of the head**
2. Oral and dental structures
3. **Nasal and sinus structures**
4. Larynx, pharynx, and guttural pouches
5. Ophthalmic structures
6. **Auricular structures**
7. Brain and nervous system
8. **Vascular anatomy**
9. Muscles
10. **Glandular structures – lymph and salivary**

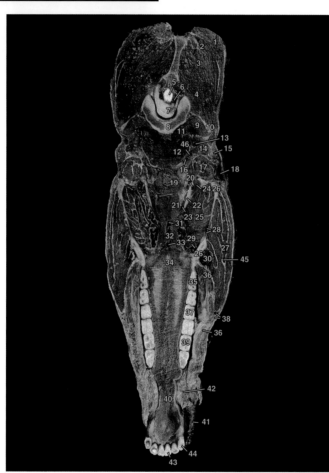

1 Splenius m.	17 Digastricus m.	33 Oropharynx
2 Rhomboideus m.	**18 Maxillary v.**	34 Intrinsic muscles of the tongue
3 Semispinalis capitis m.	19 Esophagus	**35 Tooth 311 (left third inferior molar)**
4 Obliquus capitis caudalis m.	**20 External carotid a.**	36 Buccinator m.
5 Cervical spinal cord	21 Pharyngeal mm.	**37 Tooth 309 (left first inferior molar)**
6 Ventral vertebral v.	**22 Stylohyoid bone**	**38 Facial a. and v.**
7 Body of the axis (C2)	23 Stylopharyngeus m.	**39 Tooth 307 (left third inferior premolar)**
8 Ventral arch of the atlas (C1)	24 Stylohyoideus m.	40 Genioglossus m.
9 Obliquus capitis cranialis m.	25 Medial pterygoid m.	**41 Inferior labium**
10 Wing of the atlas	**26 Mandible**	**42 Buccal salivary glands**
11 Ventral rectus capitis m.	27 Masseter m.	**43 Tooth 301 (left inferior central incisor)**
12 Longus capitis m.	**28 Inferior alveolar a. and v.**	**44 Tooth 303 (left inferior corner incisor)**
13 Occipital v.	**29 Sublingual v. branch**	**45 Masseteric v.**
14 Mandibular salivary gland	**30 Buccal venous sinus**	**46 Occipital a.**
15 Parotid salivary gland	31 Pharynx (collapsed)	
16 Internal carotid a.	32 Soft palate	

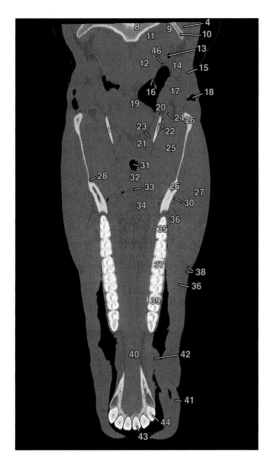

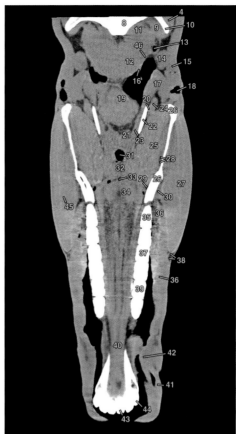

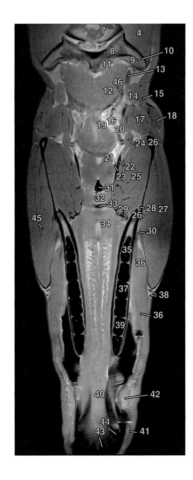

D9

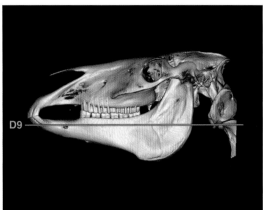

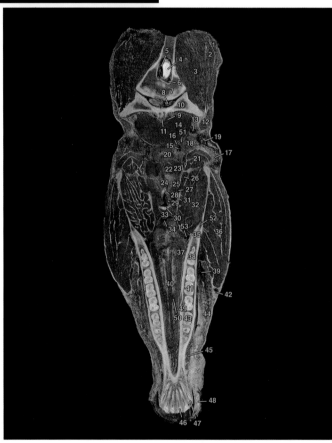

1. Bones of the head
2. Oral and dental structures
3. Nasal and sinus structures
4. Larynx, pharynx, and guttural pouches
5. Ophthalmic structures
6. Auricular structures
7. Brain and nervous system
8. Vascular anatomy
9. Muscles
10. Glandular structures – lymph and salivary

1 Splenius m.
2 Semispinalis capitis m.
3 Obliquus capitis cranialis m.
4 Cervical spinal cord
5 Dura mater
6 Ventral vertebral v.
7 Body of the axis (C2)
8 Ventral longitudinal ligament
9 Ventral rectus capitis m.
10 Ventral arch of the atlas
11 Ventral tubercle of the atlas
12 Brachiocephalicus m.
13 Occipital v.
14 Longus capitis m.
15 External carotid a. and vagosympathetic trunk
16 Internal carotid a.
17 Parotid salivary gland
18 Mandibular salivary gland

19 Maxillary v.
20 Esophagus
21 Digastricus m. (caudal belly)
22 Palatopharyngeus m.
23 Hyopharyngeus m.
24 Cricoarytenoideus dorsalis m.
25 Thyropharyngeus m.
26 Stylohyoideus m.
27 Linguofacial trunk (artery)
28 Arytenoid cartilage of the larynx, corrniculate process
29 Vocalis m.
30 Epiglottic cartilage
31 Stylohyoid bone
32 Medial pterygoid m.
33 Soft palate
34 Oropharynx
35 Body of the mandible
36 Masseter m.

37 Intrinsic muscles of the tongue
38 Tooth 311 (left inferior third molar)
39 Buccal venous sinus
40 Genioglossus m.
41 Tooth 309 (left inferior first molar)
42 Facial a. and v.
43 Tooth 307 (left inferior third premolar)
44 Buccinator m.
45 Depressor labii inferioris m.
46 Tooth 301 (left inferior central incisor)
47 Tooth 303 (left inferior corner incisor)
48 Labii inferioris
49 Mylohyoideus m.
50 Deep lingual a. and v.
51 Occipital a.
52 Inferior alveolar a. and v.
53 Sublingual v. branch

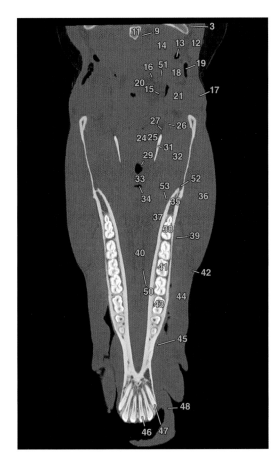

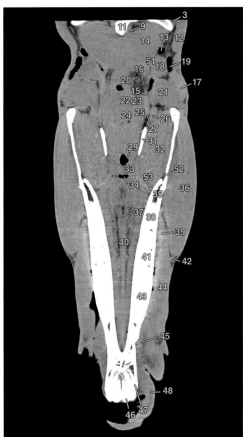

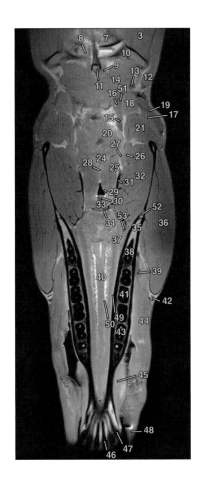

D10

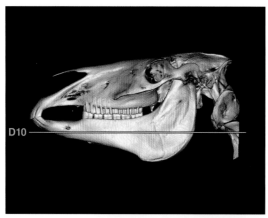

1. Bones of the head
2. Oral and dental structures
3. Nasal and sinus structures
4. Larynx, pharynx, and guttural pouches
5. Ophthalmic structures
6. Auricular structures
7. Brain and nervous system
8. Vascular anatomy
9. Muscles
10. Glandular structures – lymph and salivary

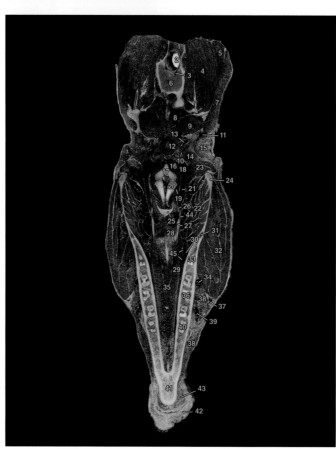

1 Dorsal lamina of the axis	17 Cricoid cartilage	33 Reserve crown of tooth 311 (left inferior third molar)
2 Cervical spinal cord	18 Cricopharyngeus m.	
3 Ventral vertebral v.	19 Ventricular m.	**34 Buccal venous sinus**
4 Obliquus capitis caudalis m.	20 Arytenoid cartilage	35 Genioglossus m.
5 Semispinalis capitis m.	21 Thyropharyngeus m.	36 Reserve crown of tooth 309 (left inferior first molar)
6 Body of the axis	22 Medial pterygoid m.	
7 Brachiocephalicus m.	23 Digastricus m. (caudal belly)	**37 Facial a. and v.**
8 Longus colli m.	**24 Caudal border of the ramus of the mandible**	38 Depressor labii inferioris m.
9 Longus capitis m.		**39 Inferior labialis v.**
10 Medial retropharyngeal lymph nodes	**25 Epiglottic cartilage**	40 Reserve crown of tooth 307 (left inferior third premolar)
11 Maxillary v.	**26 Thyroid cartilage**	
12 Esophagus	**27 Stylohyoid bone**	**41 Rostral extent of the mandible**
13 **Common carotid a.**, vagosympathetic trunk	**28 Intrinsic muscles of the tongue**	42 Orbicularis oris m.
	29 Hyoglossus m.	43 Incisivus inferioris m.
14 Mandibular salivary gland	30 Mylohyoideus m.	**44 Linguofacial trunk (a.)**
15 Parotid salivary gland	31 Inferior alveolar a., v., and n.	**45 Sublingual v. branches**
16 Cricoarytenoideus dorsalis m.	32 Masseter m.	

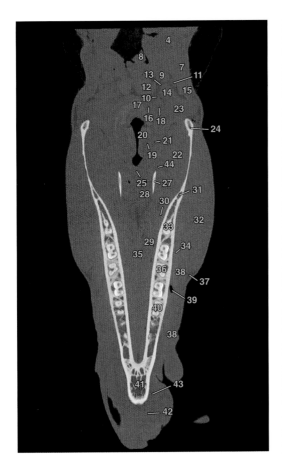

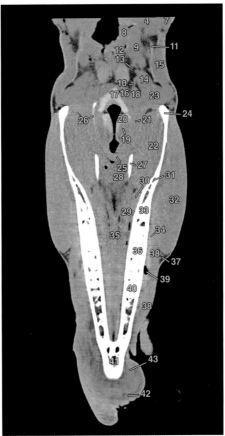

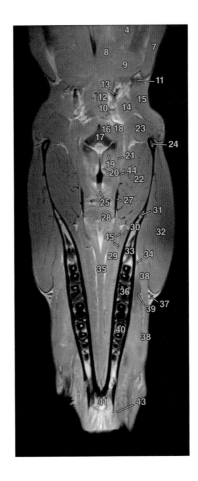

D11

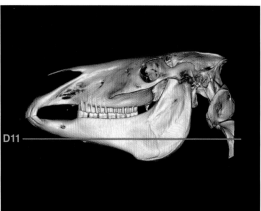

1. **Bones of the head**
2. Oral and dental structures
3. **Nasal and sinus structures**
4. Larynx, pharynx, and guttural pouches
5. Ophthalmic structures
6. **Auricular structures**
7. Brain and nervous system
8. **Vascular anatomy**
9. Muscles
10. **Glandular structures – lymph and salivary**

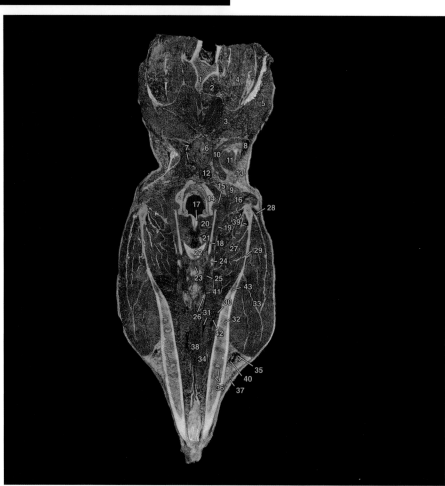

1 Ventral tubercle of the axis	16 Digastricus m.	**31 Sublingual v.**
2 Longus colli m.	17 Vocal folds	**32 Root of tooth 310 (left inferior second molar)**
3 Longus capitis m.	18 Thyroid cartilage	
4 Obliquus capitis caudalis m.	19 Thyropharyngeus m.	33 Masseter m.
5 Brachiocephalicus m.	20 Vocalis m.	34 Hyoglossus m.
6 Esophagus	21 Ventricularis m.	**35 Facial a. and v.**
7 Common carotid a.	22 Epiglottic cartilage	**36 Root of tooth 308 (left inferior fourth premolar)**
8 Maxillary v.	23 Hyoepiglotticus m.	
9 Mandibular salivary gland	**24 Thyrohyoid bone**	37 Buccinator m.
10 Sternohyoideus and omohyoideus mm.	25 Ceratohyoideus m.	38 Genioglossus m.
11 Sternocephalicus m.	**26 Ceratohyoid bone**	**39 Pterygoid branches of facial a. and v.**
12 Thyroid gland	27 Medial pterygoid m.	**40 Inferior labialis v.**
13 Parotid salivary gland	**28 Ventral masseteric v.**	**41 Lingual a.**
14 Cricoid cartilage	**29 Body of the mandible**	**42 Sublingual v. branch**
15 Cricothyroideus lateralis m.	30 Mylohyoideus m.	**43 Inferior alveolar a. and v.**

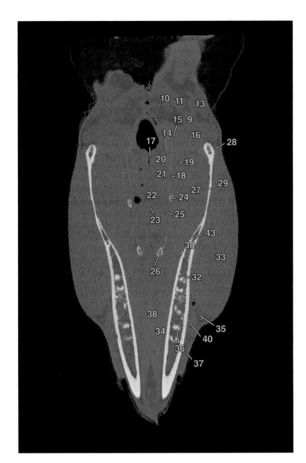

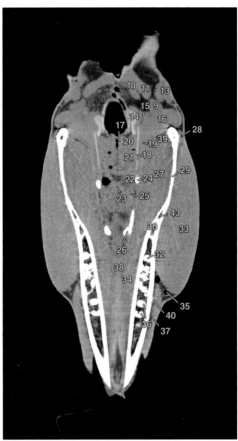

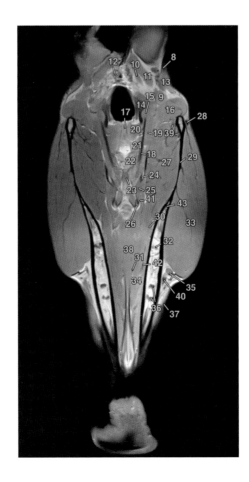

D12

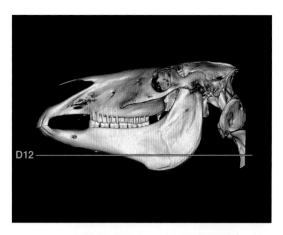

1. **Bones of the head**
2. **Oral and dental structures**
3. **Nasal and sinus structures**
4. Larynx, pharynx, and guttural pouches
5. **Ophthalmic structures**
6. **Auricular structures**
7. Brain and nervous system
8. **Vascular anatomy**
9. Muscles
10. **Glandular structures – lymph and salivary**

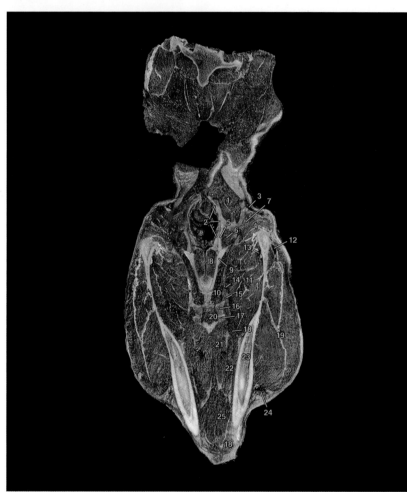

1 Longus capitis m.	10 Thyrohyoideus m.	18 Mylohyoideus m.
2 Tracheal cartilage	11 Medial pterygoid m.	19 Masseter m.
3 Maxillary v.	**12 Ventral masseteric v.**	20 Hyoepiglotticus m.
4 Digastricus m.	**13 Pterygoid branches of facial a.**	21 Hyoglossus m.
5 Cricoid cartilage	**and v.**	22 Styloglossus m.
6 Cricothyroideus m.	14 Facial a.	**23 Ramus of the mandible**
7 Mandibular salivary gland	15 Digastricus tendon	**24 Facial v. and a.**
8 Vocalis m.	**16 Thyrohyoid bone**	25 Genioglossus m.
9 Thyroid cartilage	**17 Ceratohyoid bone**	

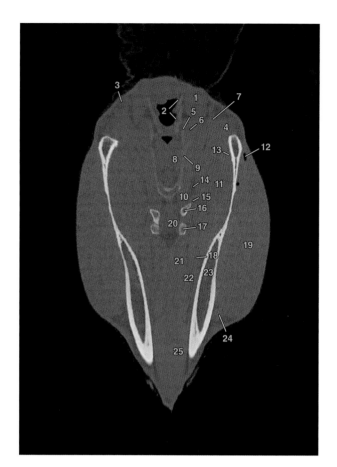

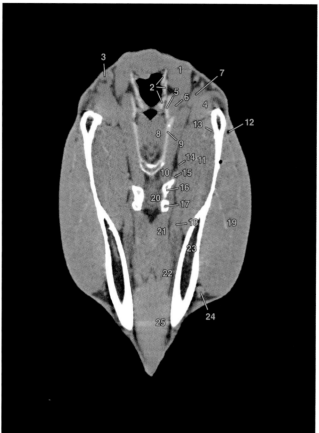

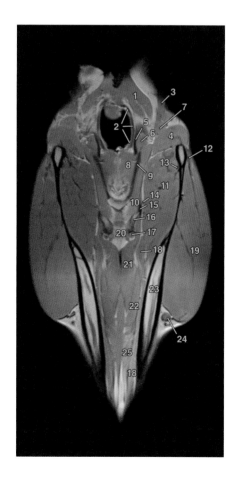

D13

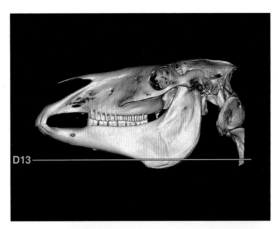

1. **Bones of the head**
2. **Oral and dental structures**
3. **Nasal and sinus structures**
4. Larynx, pharynx, and guttural pouches
5. **Ophthalmic structures**
6. **Auricular structures**
7. Brain and nervous system
8. **Vascular anatomy**
9. Muscles
10. **Glandular structures – lymph and salivary**

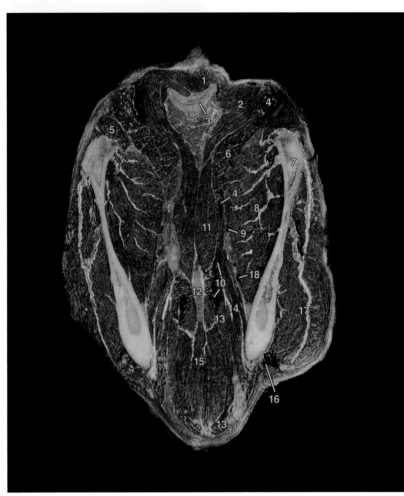

1 Sternohyoideus m.	**7 Mandible**	13 Mylohyoideus m.
2 Omohyoideus m.	8 Medial pterygoid m.	14 Digastricus m. (rostral belly)
3 Tracheal ring	**9 Sublingual a.**	15 Geniohyoideus m.
4 Linguofacial v.	**10 Lingual v.**	**16 Facial a. and v.**
5 Digastricus m.	11 Omohyoideus and sternohyoideus mm.	17 Masseter m.
6 Mandibular salivary gland	**12 Lingual process of basihyoid bone**	**18 Facial a.**

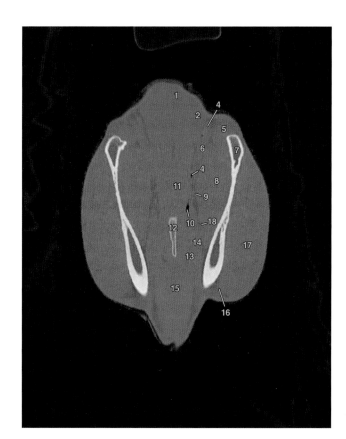

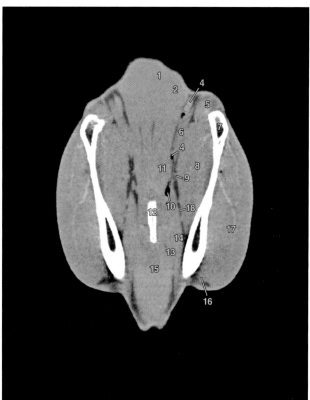

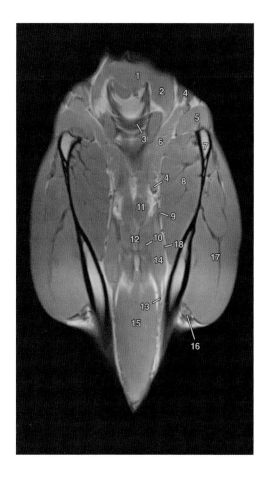

Glossary

Directional terms

Anterior – in bipeds, anterior refers to the surface of the body towards the belly and corresponds to the term "ventral" used in quadrupeds. In quadrupeds, its use is limited to structures of the eye and inner ear.

Axial – used distal to the carpus and tarsus. It refers to the surface facing the axis of the limb, which in multidigited animals is defined as passing between the third and fourth digits. The opposite surface is described as the abaxial surface.

Buccal – formerly used to refer to the surface of the tooth adjacent to the cheek; the vestibular surface of the premolars and molars.

Caudal – toward or relatively closer to the tail. This term is used of the neck, trunk, limbs, and head.

Cranial – towards or relatively closer to the head. This term is used of the neck, trunk, and limbs only.

Distal – relatively further from the main body mass or the origin; on the teeth, it is the surface of the tooth that is adjacent to the more caudal or lateral tooth.

Dorsal – towards or relatively closer to the back or vertebral column; corresponds to "posterior" in bipeds. This term is used on the head, neck, and trunk. On the limbs, it refers to the surface of the manus and pes opposite the surface with the pads.

External – closer to the superficial surface.

Inferior – in bipeds, this term refers to structures further from the head. In veterinary medicine, its use is limited to structures associated with the lips and teeth.

Internal – further from the external surface.

Labial – formerly used to refer to the surface of the teeth facing the lips; it is the vestibular surface of the incisors.

Lateral – further from the median plane (a plane drawn through the midline of the body that divides it into equal right and left parts).

Lingual – towards the tongue; refers to the surface of the teeth facing the tongue.

Medial – closer to the median plane (a plane drawn through the midline of the body that divides it into equal right and left parts).

Mesial – surface of a tooth toward the midline or adjacent to the next rostral or medial tooth.

Posterior – in bipeds, it refers to the surface of the body closer to the back or vertebral column. It corresponds to the term "dorsal" that is used in quadrupeds. Its use in quadrupeds is limited to some structures of the eye and ear.

Sagittal plane – a plane drawn through the long axis of the body or an organ that divides it into right and left parts.

Superior – in bipeds, refers to structures closer to the head. Its use in quadrupeds is limited to structures associated with the lips.

Transverse plane – a plane drawn through the body that divides it into cranial and caudal parts.

Ventral – towards or relatively nearer the belly.

Vestibular – the surface of the tooth that faces away from the tongue and towards the lips or cheeks.

Anatomical and imaging terms

Algorithm – step-by-step procedure used by computers to solve mathematical problems.

Basal – towards the base.

Cochlea – spiral form; resembling a snail.

Concha – structure or part that resembles a shell.

Condyle – a rounded articular projection on a bone.

Coronoid – hooked or curved; resembling a crown.

CT – computed tomography.

Diverticulum – a circumscribed pouch or sac.

Epi – upon.

Ethmoid – sieve-like.

FLAIR (MRI) – inversion recovery is a type of MR sequence, and can null the signal from either fluid (fluid attenuation inversion recovery or FLAIR) or fat (short-tau inversion recovery or STIR). The FLAIR sequence is useful to differentiate pure fluid from proteinaceous fluid, and to better define the margins of a fluid-filled space or pocket.

Foramen – a natural opening or passageway through a bone.

Greater – the larger of two similar structures.

Hemi – one half.

Hounsfield unit – CT uses a method of attenuation to display an image by converting a volume of tissue to a three-dimensional pixel called a voxel. CT will determine the average linear attenuation coefficient of X-rays for each voxel in a patient at a particular location. Each voxel can be given a quantifiable number in terms of its gray scale, termed a Hounsfield unit. As a reference, pure water has a HU of 0 and air is −1000 HU.

Hyo – shaped like a lower-case Greek letter upsilon (υ). In the head, it refers to structures associated with the hyoid apparatus.

Hypo – under or below.

Infra – below or beneath.

Isotropic – similar in all directions.

Labium – fleshy border or edge; on the head, it refers to the lip.

Lacrimal – pertaining to tears.

Lesser – the smaller of two similar structures.

Lingual – associated with the tongue.

Major – the larger of two similar structures.

Meatus – opening or passageway.

Minor – the smaller of two similar structures.

MRI – magnetic resonance imaging.

Myo – associated with or having to do with muscle.

Atlas of Clinical Imaging and Anatomy of the Equine Head, First Edition. Larry Kimberlin, Alex zur Linden and Lynn Ruoff.
© 2017 John Wiley & Sons, Inc. Published 2017 by John Wiley & Sons, Inc.

Nasal – associated with the nose.

Nuchal – referring to the dorsal surface of the neck.

Omo – associated with the shoulder.

Palatine – pertaining to the palate.

Palpebral – referring to the eyelids.

Parietal – referring to the wall.

Parotid – situated close to the ear.

Petrous – resembling a rock.

Pineal – shaped like a pine cone.

Piriform – pear-shaped.

Pixel – the smallest element of an image that can be individually processed in a video display system.

Rectus – straight.

Retro – backward or behind.

Rugae – folds or wrinkles.

Semi – one-half; partly.

Septum – dividing wall or partition.

Sinus – space; in the head, it refers to air-filled spaces in some of the bones of the skull.

Spinous – resembling a thorn.

Squamous – scale-like, flattened.

STIR (MRI) – inversion recovery is a type of MR sequence, and can null the signal from either fluid (fluid attenuation inversion recovery or FLAIR) or fat (short-tau inversion recovery or STIR). The STIR sequence is useful to identify pathology (inflammation, edema) without mistaking it for hyperintense fat.

Stylo – resembling a stylus; pointed.

Sub – under or below.

Super, supra – above.

Tubercle – a rounded bony prominence.

T weighting (MRI) – radiofrequency energy is absorbed by the protons in the body and emitted at certain rates (T2 and T1 relaxation). There are multiple different types of MR sequences that can be performed, and for the most part they are related to timing differences of the emitted energy from the protons, or relaxation times. These sequences include T2 weighted, T1 weighted, T2* weighted, proton density (PD), and inversion recovery (fat or fluid suppression).

Tympanic – resembling a drum; air filled.

Vomer – cutting blade of a plow.

Voxel – a three-dimensional pixel.

Window level (WL)/window width (WW) – the computer uses an algorithm or filter to adjust how each pixel looks on a two-dimensional image and this algorithm can be modified to alter the spatial resolution and contrast differences of different tissues. The primary two algorithms used in this book are referred to generically as a bone filter or algorithm and a soft tissue filter or algorithm. The bone algorithm has a higher spatial resolution and the bone and teeth are seen in gray with well-defined edges, whereas all of the soft tissues are homogenously gray. The soft tissue algorithm has a reduced spatial resolution but the contrast of the soft tissues is more noticeable, and the bone and teeth are completely white. The appearance of the CT images can be adjusted by the viewer for either algorithm using the window width/window level adjustment function found on all image-viewing systems. The window width (WW) is the range of displayed Hounsfield units. The window level (WL) is the Hounsfield unit in the center of the window width.

Zygo – yoked or paired.

References

Articles

Arencibia A, Vazquez JM, Jaber R, *et al.* (2000) Magnetic resonance imaging and cross-sectional anatomy of the normal equine sinuses and nasal passages. *Veterinary Radiology and Ultrasound*, **41** (4), 313–319.

Goncalves R, Malalana F, McConnell JF, Maddox T (2015) Anatomical study of cranial nerve emergency and skull foramina in the horse using magnetic resonance imaging and computed tomography. *Veterinary Radiology and Ultrasound*, **56** (4), 391–397.

Morrow KL, Park RD, Spurgeon TL, Stashak TS, Arceneaux B (2000) Computed tomographic imaging of the equine head. *Veterinary Radiology and Ultrasound*, **41** (6), 491–497.

Probst A, Henninger W, Willmann M (2005) Communications of normal nasal and paranasal cavities in computed tomography of horses. *Veterinary Radiology and Ultrasound*, **46** (1), 44–48.

Rodriguez MJ, Latorre R, Lopez-Albors O, *et al.* (2008) Computed tomographic anatomy of the temporomandibular joint in the young horse. *Equine Veterinary Journal*, **40** (6), 561–571.

Rodriguez MJ, Agut A, Soler M, *et al.* (2010) Magnetic resonance imaging of the equine temporomandibular joint anatomy. *Equine Veterinary Journal*, **42** (3), 200–207.

Books

Ashdown RR, Done SH (2011) *Color Atlas of Veterinary Anatomy*, vol. 2. Mosby/Elsevier, Philadelphia, PA.

Budras KD, Sack WO, Rock S (2003) *Anatomy of the Horse*. Schlutersche, Hanover, Germany.

Dyce KM, Sack WO, Wensing CJ (2010) *Textbook of Veterinary Anatomy*. Saunders/Elsevier, Philadelphia, PA.

Getty R (1975) *Sisson and Grossman's The Anatomy of the Domestic Animals*. WB Saunders, Philadelphia, PA.

International Committee on Veterinary Gross Anatomical Nomenclature (2012) *Nomina Anatomica Veterinaria*. World Association of Veterinary Anatomists, Knoxville, TN.

Konig HE, Liebich HG (eds) (2007) *Veterinary Anatomy of Domestic Mammals*, 3rd edn. Schattauer, Stuttgart, Germany.

Murray RC (ed.) (2011) *Equine MRI*. Wiley-Blackwell, Oxford, UK.

Popesko P (1977) *Atlas of Topographical Anatomy of the Domestic Animals*, vol. 1, 2nd edn. WB Saunders, Philadelphia, PA.

Schaller O (ed.) (2007) *Illustrated Veterinary Anatomical Nomenclature*, 2nd edn. Enke, Stuttgart, Germany.

Index

Atlas of Clinical Imaging and Anatomy of the Equine Head, First Edition. Larry Kimberlin, Alex zur Linden and Lynn Ruoff.
© 2017 John Wiley & Sons, Inc. Published 2017 by John Wiley & Sons, Inc.